IMAGES
of America

SANATORIUMS OF NEW MEXICO

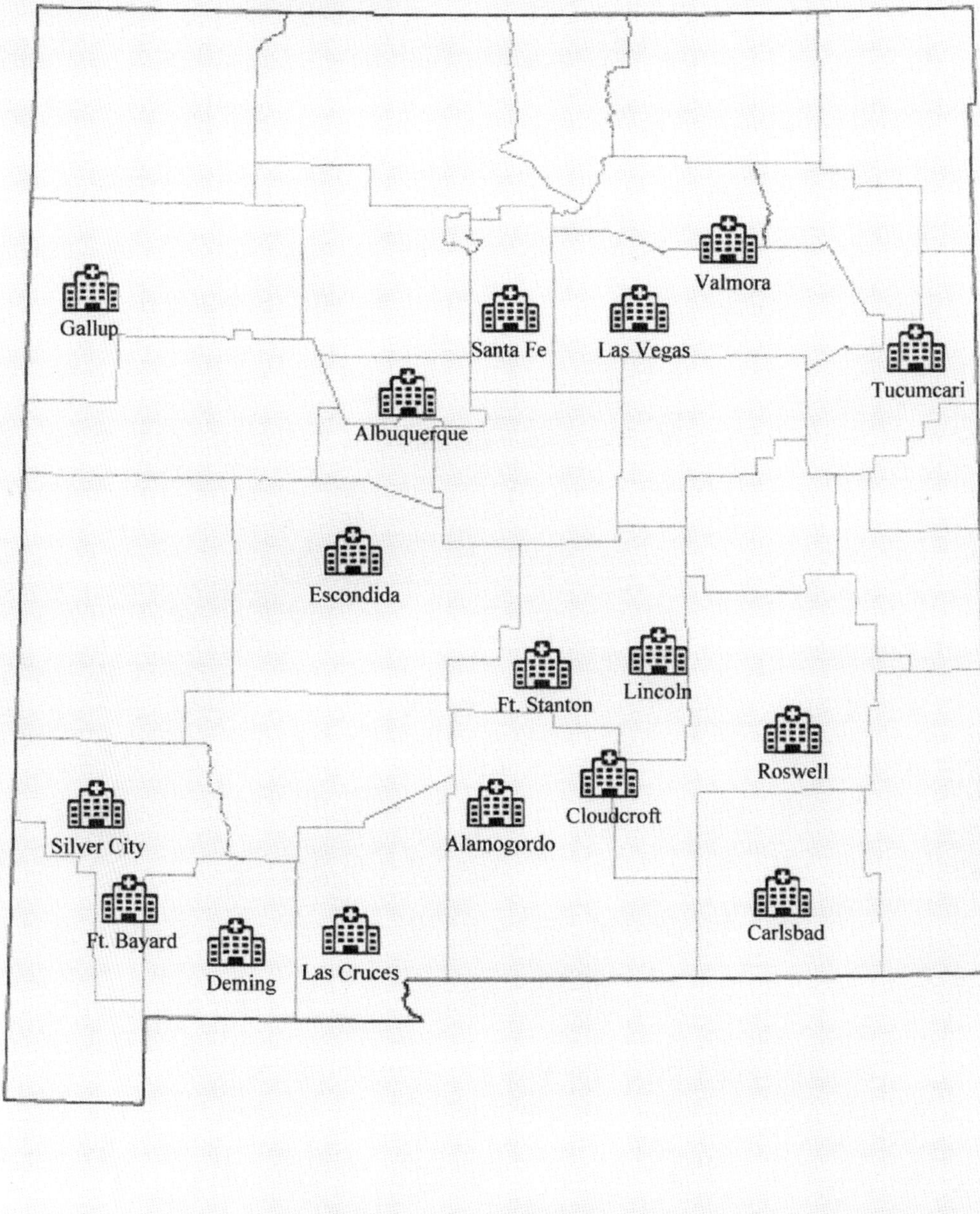

This map shows New Mexico communities with well-known tuberculosis sanatoriums between 1865 and 1970. (Courtesy of Baldwin G. Burr.)

On the Cover: The Presbyterian Sanatorium in Albuquerque, New Mexico, is shown about 1967. (Courtesy of Presbyterian Healthcare Services.)

IMAGES
of America

SANATORIUMS OF NEW MEXICO

Richard Melzer
Foreword by Jake W. Spidle Jr.

ARCADIA
PUBLISHING

ISBN 978-1-4671-3132-2

Published by Arcadia Publishing
Charleston, South Carolina

Printed in the United States of America

Library of Congress Control Number: 2013957644

For all general information, please contact Arcadia Publishing:
Telephone 843-853-2070
Fax 843-853-0044
E-mail sales@arcadiapublishing.com
For customer service and orders:
Toll-Free 1-888-313-2665

Visit us on the Internet at www.arcadiapublishing.com

To Jessica Mack, MD, our truly amazing daughter-in-law

Contents

Foreword

When I finished turning the last few pages of Professor Melzer's wonderful *Sanatoriums of New Mexico*, I had one of those smack-yourself-flush-in-the-forehead moments. Why in the world had I not thought to do a book such as this? Compact, visually compelling, and strikingly accessible, it is a most palatable overview of a critically important piece of New Mexico's recent past. Frankly speaking, I am not just impressed, but also more than a little jealous of Melzer's remarkable success with this book.

Second thoughts, however, suggest it is probably better that this contribution was left to him. There are few writer-researchers around who have contributed more to the modern-day study of New Mexico history than he. In both quantity and quality, it is hard to think of many, or any, historians of our present-day generation who have added more to our understanding of New Mexico's past. In his historical ramblings, he has ranged back into the Spanish and Mexican periods of this region's history and culture, but he has been most at home ransacking the recesses of 20th-century New Mexico's past—the Civilian Conservation Corps; atom-bomb spying in 1940s Los Alamos; Madrid as an exemplar of New Mexico's mining culture; Harvey Houses and their role in creating a modern tourism industry; Ernie Pyle; gravesites; childhood in the West; Valencia County history. All of these topics have been so usefully and productively spread across his worktable. I can think of no one who has more thoroughly and broadly examined the cupboards and closets, highways and byways of New Mexico's modern history than Professor Melzer.

This new book adds importantly to Melzer's impressive body of work and to a more comprehensive, fuller understanding of the 20th century in this faraway place. In a graceful and eye-catching way, he puts the final touches to one of the most important developments within the recent study of New Mexico's history—the "discovery" of the roles of tuberculosis and the tuberculosis industry in the making of modern New Mexico. If a reader examines the basic textbooks and general surveys of the region's past from the 1940s, 1950s, and 1960s, a strong consensus regarding the major themes of this area's modern history is evident. Virtually all the historians agreed that territorial New Mexico's development and that of the first 25 years or so of the new state of New Mexico were shaped in a fundamental way by three essential industries—ranching, railroading, and mining. But the last two generations or so of New Mexico's 20th-century historians have firmly established a fourth economic and cultural engine alongside those earlier three: the health industry associated with the arrival of many thousands of health-seekers, or lungers, as they called themselves. Touching every corner of the territory/state and impacting all aspects of its culture, economy, and social structure, the lungers—involuntary New Mexicans—are an indelible part of the shaping of late-19th and 20th-century New Mexico.

This new book by Melzer may stand as a kind of capstone to this historiographical phenomenon. He has thoroughly digested all the relevant literature, critically evaluated it, and added the weight of his own insights on the subject. So far, so good. Who better to survey and generalize than this student of modern New Mexico's heritage? Uniquely among the students of the lungers and their place in New Mexico history, Melzer has taken the time and trouble to photo-document it. He has sought out and sorted through thousands of images left to us from the world of the tuberculars to help us understand that world, until now inaccessible to us. The cliché insists that a picture is worth a thousand words. Whether or not that is really true, it is certainly true that a carefully guided visual tour through a landscape and style of life now distant and alien to us can help us develop a sympathy and level of understanding of a past reality not available in any other way.

And we can confidently trust our guide. His energy, tenacity, and good judgment in the research process have produced a harvest of material never previously pulled together in one place. As I admiringly peeled through the dozens of photographs, postcards, newspaper articles, and other images selected by Melzer for this volume, I could not escape the impression that he has seen *every* photo-document still extant illustrating this facet of New Mexico's past. That cannot be literally true, of course, but there can be no question of the thoroughness of Professor Melzer's search for just the right images to tell the tuberculosis story. He's been through all the conventional repositories that historians check, many of them on repeated visits. But even more, he has had the imagination and energy to prospect in unconventional places. Your great-aunt Adele's three scrapbooks of family photos? Yes, Professor Melzer borrowed them from her two summers ago. Those four rusting, 1940s file cabinets standing forlornly in a basement corner of the Quay County courthouse? Yep, Melzer went through them in 2009.

And the results of all that prospecting are abundantly obvious in the many arresting and never-before-published photo-documents that decorate this volume. What a painless and fascinating way to learn something important about our society's history: to see it with one's own eyes and to be guided along the way by the information and insights of a first-class storyteller and historian. In this book, the images so carefully selected allow us to see with our own eyes the everyday reality of life in the rarified world of the tuberculars. We can see, measure, and feel the physical structures of their world—the tents, sleeping porches, convalescent rooms, and the often poignantly simple, spare sanatorium rooms that were the spatial parameters of their world. Through the images, we can get a clear sense of the routines that ordered and defined their daily existence. We can see and seek to understand the tangible objects they handled and trusted, the adjuncts to the specialized daily living so unique to their lifestyles. These visual artifacts of the health-seekers' hegiras to and through this particular place at a, medically speaking, quite specific time in the long history of tuberculosis, Professor Melzer has sought out, carefully selected, and organized to help us at least partially recapture this now temporally distant part of our New Mexico heritage. And he is always so usefully at our elbow, explaining the manifold messages of the images. Through his learning (lightly worn), he helps us to see what might otherwise remain hidden.

As noted at the beginning of this foreword, I wish this book were mine, and I heartily commend it alike to professional historians and amateur students of New Mexico's past. To open it up, even at random, and scan its pages is to see and begin to fathom a 50-year piece of the New Mexico past not available anywhere else in just this way, and for that service, we are in Professor Melzer's debt.

—Jake W. Spidle Jr.

ACKNOWLEDGMENTS

A large army of incredibly helpful historians, archivists, and librarians assisted in the writing of this brief history of TB sanatoriums in New Mexico. Fellow historians included Cecilia Bell, Susan Berry, Doc Campbell, Ann Carson, Gary Cozzens, Peter Eidenbach, David Kammer, Ruth Luckasson, Liz Miskos, Nancy Owen Lewis, Katherine M. Pomonis, Kristen Reynolds, Lucinda Sachs, Dorothy A. Simpson, John Taylor, Bob White, and Jeanne Whitehouse. Archivists and librarians included Connie Clark at the Tularosa Basin Historical Museum; E. Glenn Fye at the Albuquerque Museum; Patricia Hewitt at the Museum of New Mexico; Linda Moore at the Tucumcari Historical Museum; Cynthia Shetter at the Los Lunas Museum of Heritage and Arts; Beth Silbergleit and Nancy Brown-Martinez at the Center for Southwest Research, University of New Mexico; Mo Palmer of Presbyterian Healthcare Services; Joyce Raizen and Laurie Volkin of the Lovelace Heath System; Janet Williams of the Presbyterian Medical Library; Terry Gugliotta at the University of New Mexico Archives; Janet H. Johnson and Laura J. Hall of Special Collections at the University of New Mexico's Health Science Library; Barbara Rodriguez, Judy Marquez, Esther Shir, LeAnn Weller, and Lisa Pate at the University of New Mexico–Valencia Campus library; and Lynn Shakespeare and Joan Bigben at the Albuquerque Indian Hospital. Dorothy A. Simpson kindly reviewed the section on Valmora, Gary Cozzens read the section on Fort Stanton, Kristen Reynolds read the section on Albuquerque sans, Cecilia Bell read the section on Fort Bayard, and Mo Palmer and Rena Chávez Melzer read the entire manuscript and offered many helpful suggestions. Special thanks go to Nancy Tucker, Jim Coad, Dorothy A. Simpson, Donna Henderson, Penny Hobbie, Jane Bardal, Katherine M. Pomonis, Charles Kohlass, Jeff Snodgrass at the Immaculate Heart of Mary Retreat Conference Center, the Socorro Historical Society, the Lovelace Health System, and Presbyterian Healthcare Services for generously sharing their priceless postcards and photographs. Baldwin G. Burr provided his unsurpassed technical skills.

Unless otherwise noted, all images are from the author's collection.

One

Inventing the Sans

Millions of men and women had died of tuberculosis (TB) by the middle of the 19th century. So many had succumbed to the dreaded disease that it was thought to be incurable. Some people, however, were not willing to give up so easily. Early doctors attempted bloodletting, vomiting, sweating, and other extreme measures that weakened their patients and no doubt exacerbated the disease more often than arresting it.

Later physicians prescribed "heroic treatments," urging patients to engage in such vigorous activities as hiking, mountain climbing, horseback riding, and manual labor. By 1910, Dr. Francis T.B. Fest wrote that "roughing it" in these ways had killed thousands and that, if the "foolish belief" continued, it would surely kill thousands more. Other patients were deceived by unscrupulous manufacturers of patented medicines who promised that their bogus concoctions could cure most anything, including TB.

Fortunately, saner minds prevailed, suggesting that extended periods of rest would be the best possible cure, especially in combination with mountain air, proper diets, and careful medical supervision. Sanatoriums were first established in Europe. In the United States, Dr. Edward L. Trudeau created the first successful sanatorium after realizing the benefits of such conditions in his own recovery from TB. Trudeau's Adirondack Cottage Sanatorium became the prototype for sanitariums (health resorts), or sanatoriums (hospitals specializing in TB), especially in the American Southwest. Often used interchangeably, both sanitariums and sanatoriums were commonly known as "sans."

Thousands of TB patients (also known as lungers) migrated to New Mexico, especially with the coming of the railroad to the territory in 1880. Affluent "health travelers" frequented the territory's famous health spas. Those with limited resources stayed in tents, shacks, and boardinghouses. In most cases, only those who could afford six- to nine-month stays in New Mexico's new sanatoriums could hope to survive. Sanatoriums, including the 55 facilities in New Mexico, had become the modern, medically endorsed panacea that thousands were eager to accept as their best, last hope for recovery.

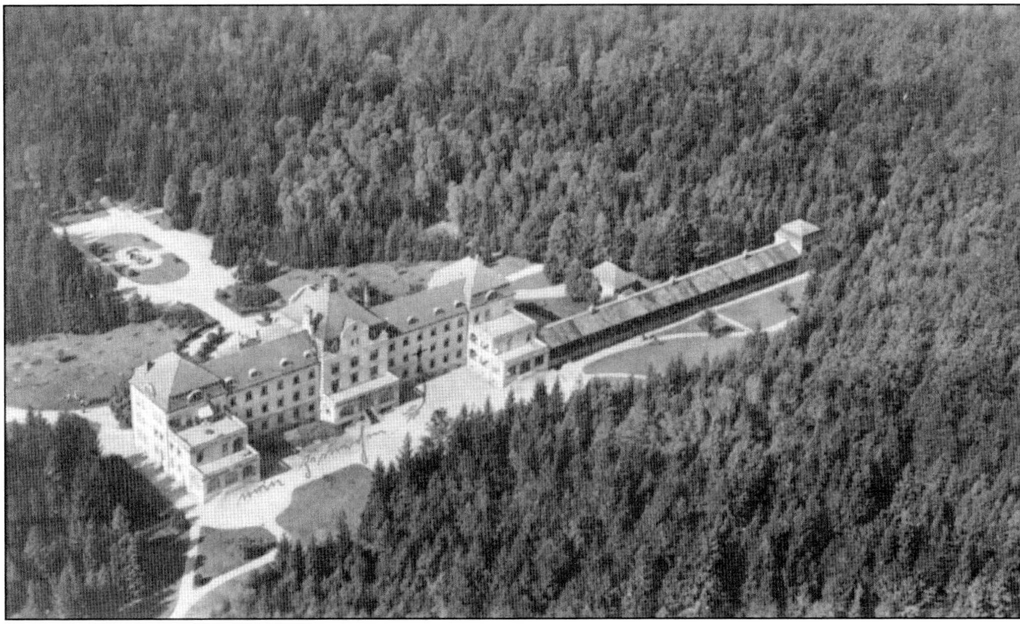

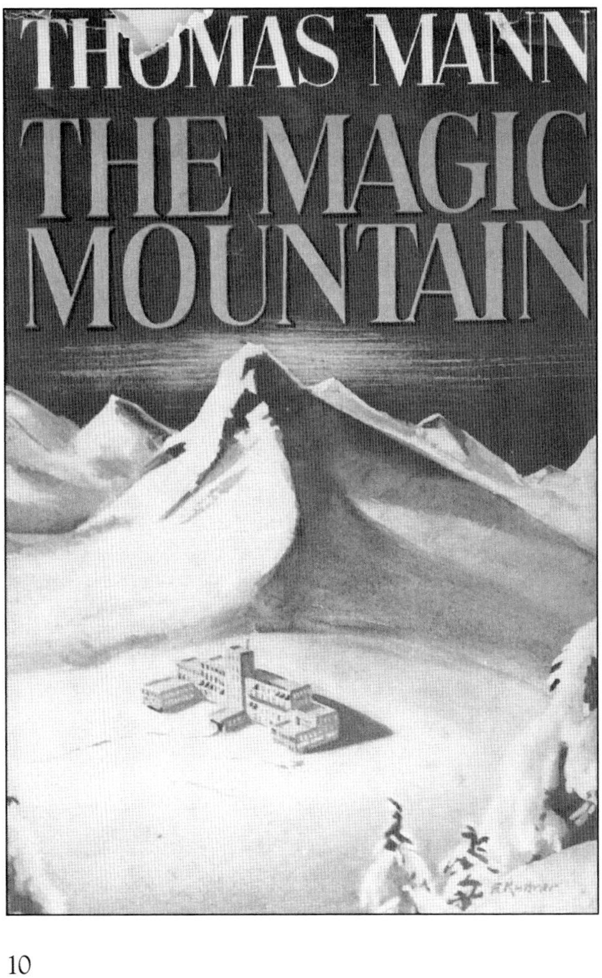

European physicians made the first attempt to treat tuberculosis with institutional care in 1854, when Dr. Hermann Brehmer established his "closed institution" at Gorbersdorf, Germany. Catering to the affluent, Brehmer's facility emphasized the value of rich food, restricted physical exercise, and clean mountain air. Dr. Peter Dettweiler took Brehmer's concepts a step further by stressing the need for direct medical supervision. Emulating this approach, doctors opened sanatoriums in many parts of Europe, especially Switzerland and Germany (pictured above). Thomas Mann's novel *The Magic Mountain* (1927) was set in one such exclusive san in the Swiss Alps. Dr. Paul Kretzschmar, a Dettweiler disciple, is given credit for introducing his mentor's ideas in the United States by the 1880s. The sanatorium movement in America had begun.

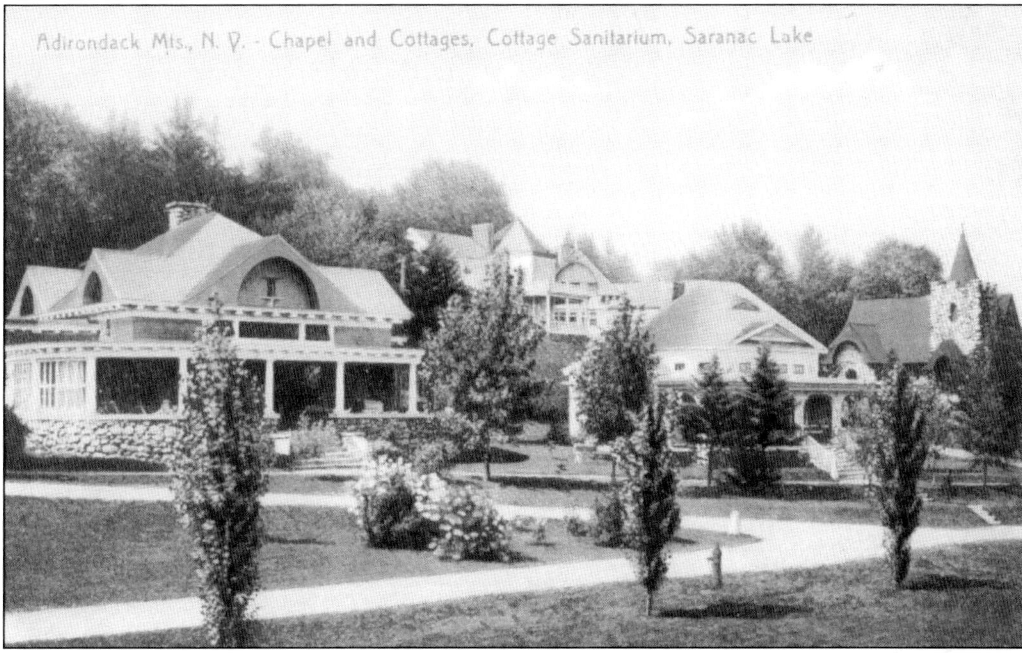
Adirondack Mts., N. Y. - Chapel and Cottages, Cottage Sanitarium, Saranac Lake

While other doctors attempted to establish the first sanatoriums in the United States (specifically in North Carolina), Dr. Edward L. Trudeau was the first to enjoy lasting success. Like so many other TB specialists, he had first recovered from the disease before entering the field himself. Living in the Adirondack Mountains when doctors gave him little chance of recovery, Trudeau became convinced that rest, diet, exposure to clean, thin air, and sound medical care were key elements in restoring a TB patient's health. Opened in 1884, his famous san, with its private, individual cottages at Saranac Lake, New York, became the model for sans across the country, including New Mexico. Respected physicians, including Dr. Carl Mulky and Dr. Carl Gellenthien of New Mexico, made annual visits to Saranac Lake to learn the latest techniques in Trudeau's "cottage cure."

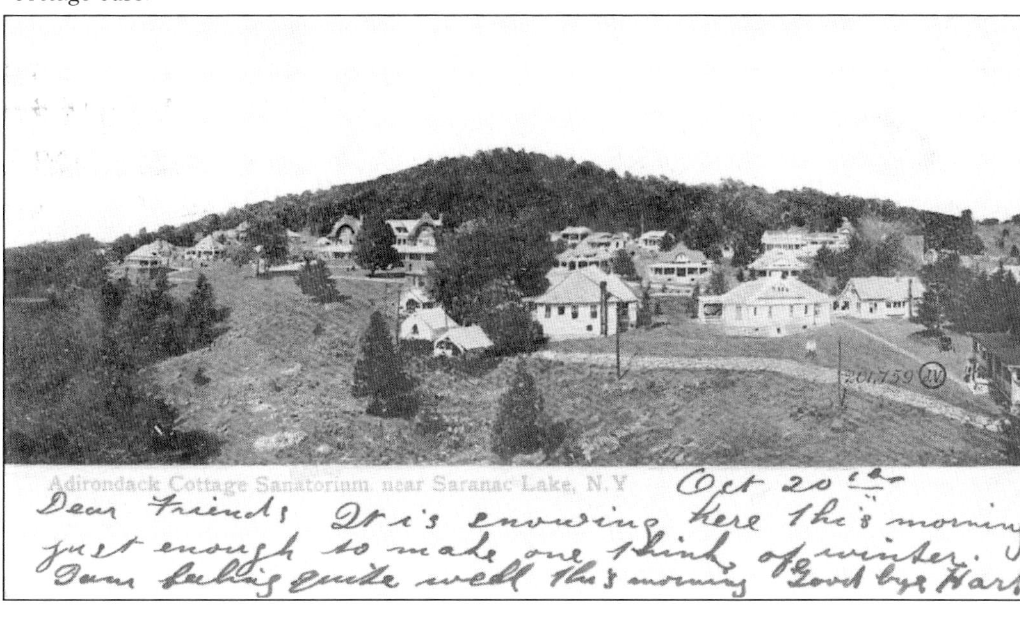
201759
Adirondack Cottage Sanatorium near Saranac Lake, N.Y
Oct 20th
Dear Friend; It is snowing here this morning
just enough to make one think of winter.
I am feeling quite well this morning Good bye Hart

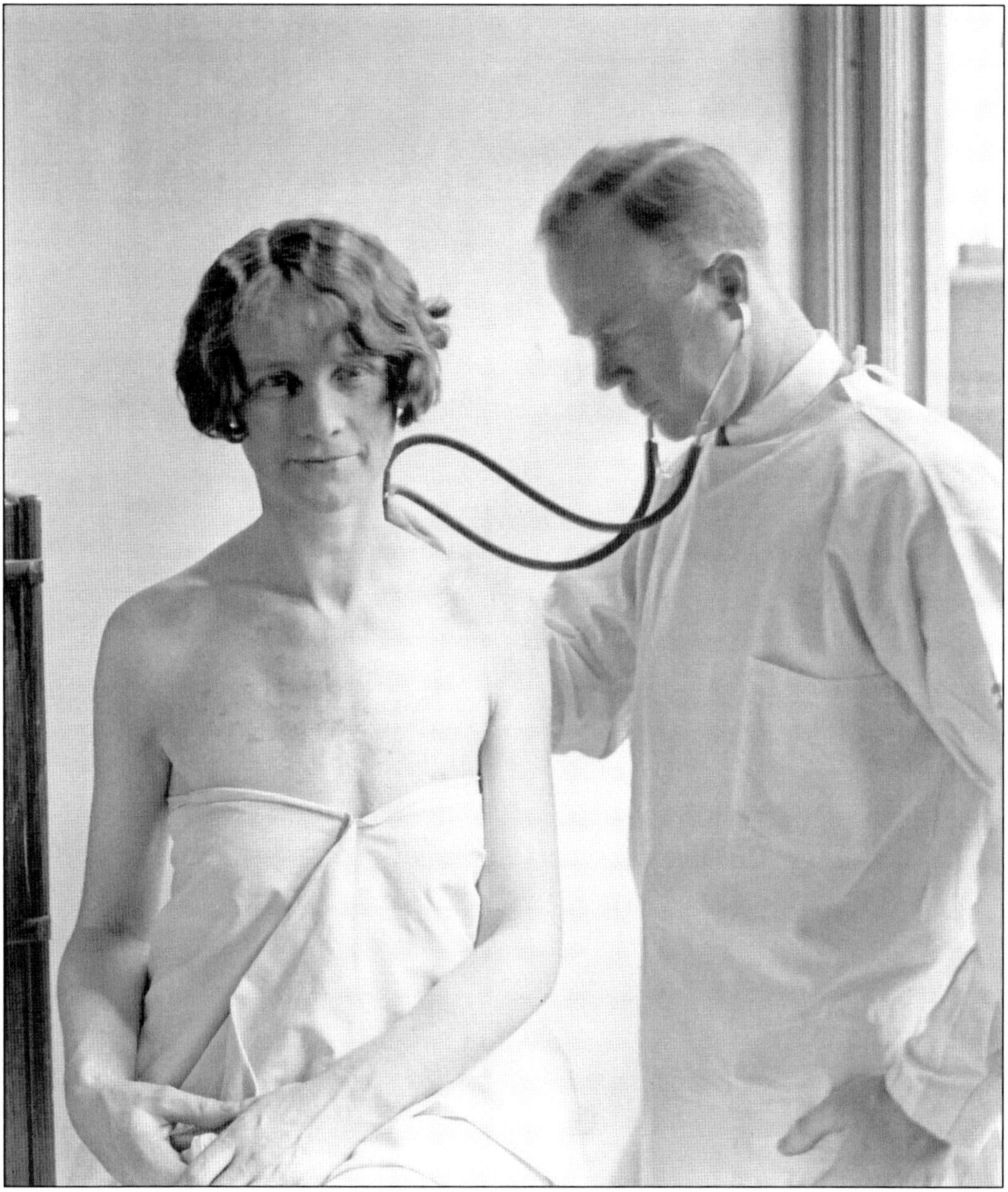

Lungers received the "terrible truth" of their disease after lung examinations and chest X-rays by their regular physicians and, in many cases, TB experts. Most victims came to New Mexico from the Midwest, especially states like Illinois, Ohio, and Indiana. Others came from abroad, especially Canada and Great Britain. A survey of Fairview Cemetery records in Albuquerque shows that the 693 lungers who were buried at the graveyard from 1881 to 1920 had been engaged in at least 41 different jobs or professions, ranging from the traditional (teachers, lawyers, and clerks) to the unusual, including a matchmaker, a gambler, and a steamboat captain. Marriage was postponed temporarily or permanently for many young men and women in sans. According to the Fairview survey, single lungers outnumbered married ones, six to one. With so much of their lives interrupted, it was as if lungers served prison terms for crimes they did not commit, with a probation that carried social stigma long after their "release."

Playing on the national fear of tuberculosis, newspapers and magazines were filled with advertisements claiming "surefire" methods to both prevent and cure the disease. Even credible products like Listerine (right) professed to prevent TB by destroying germs in general. Most other preventions and "cures" were far less believable. Piso's Cure (below) sold widely, although its advertisements told consumers that "you must not ask us to reveal [our] valuable secrets." When its chicanery was exposed, Piso's Cure was found to include cannabis (marijuana), chloroform, and alcohol, ingredients that undermined rather than cured TB. New medical "discoveries" were reported almost daily, making it difficult for consumers to separate fact from fiction. In 1919, the National Tuberculosis Association reported that, of more than 500 "medical concoctions" on the market, "not one of them has been found to be even partly successful" in curing TB.

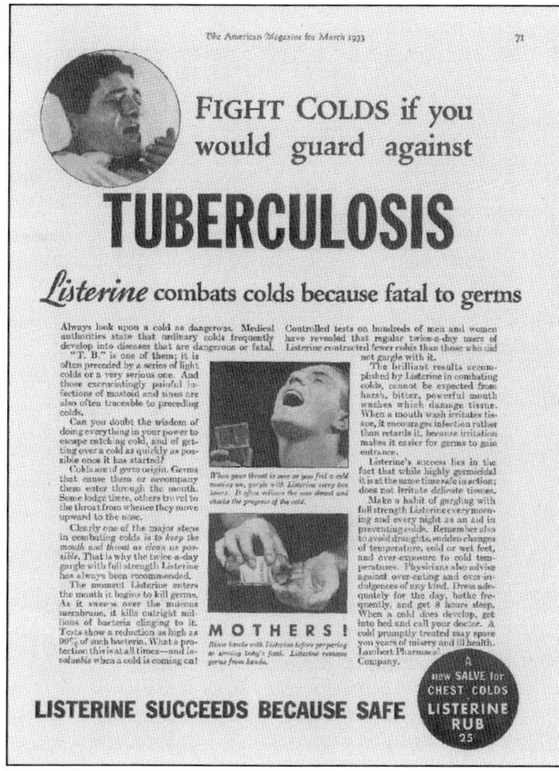

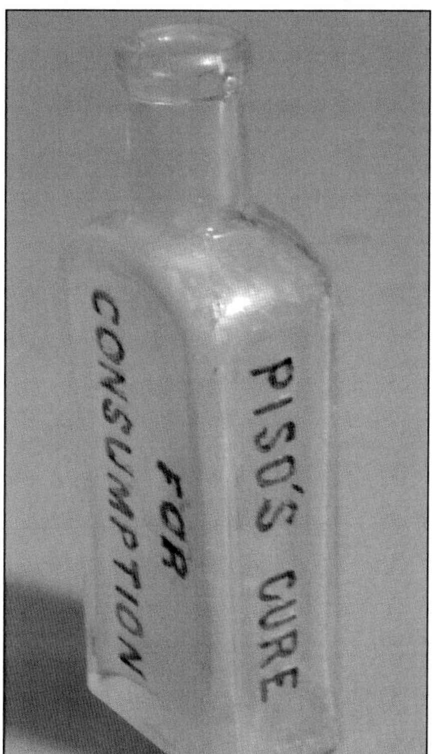

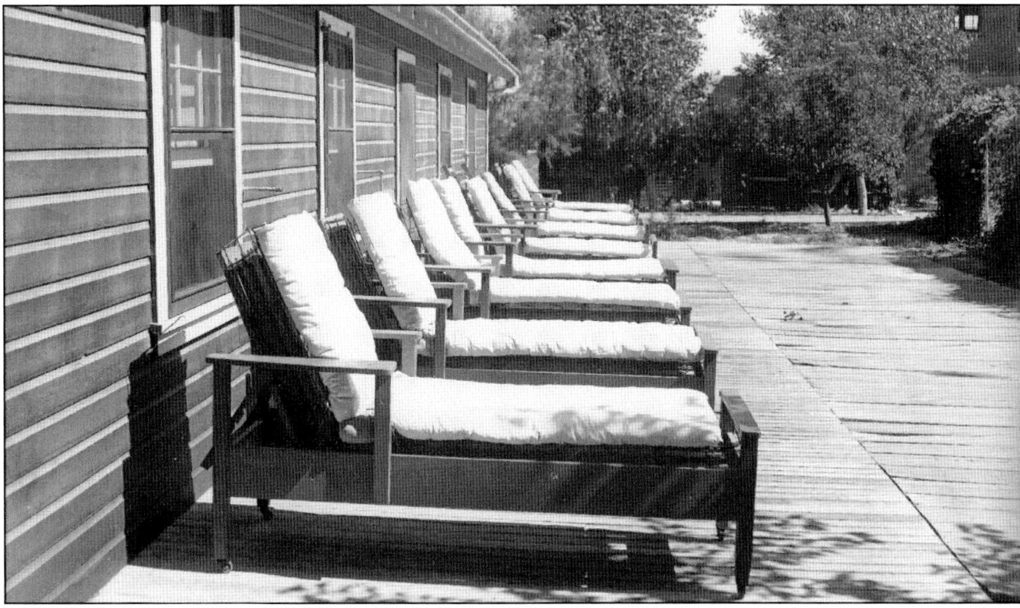

TB patients were expected to spend as much as seven to twelve hours of their day outside, breathing the clean, fresh air they had come to New Mexico to enjoy. Although New Mexico's climate was mild compared to other states and superior to any part of the world, if booster literature was to be believed, most of the state had its share of cold temperatures, snow, and high winds. Lungers soon learned the important skill of wrapping themselves in blankets for maximum warmth while sitting outdoors on lounge chairs in cold weather. Of course, blankets were shed in New Mexico's extreme summer heat, which allowed for another popular form of treatment: heliotherapy, or simple sunbathing. (Above, courtesy of the Albuquerque Museum, PA1992.5.460.)

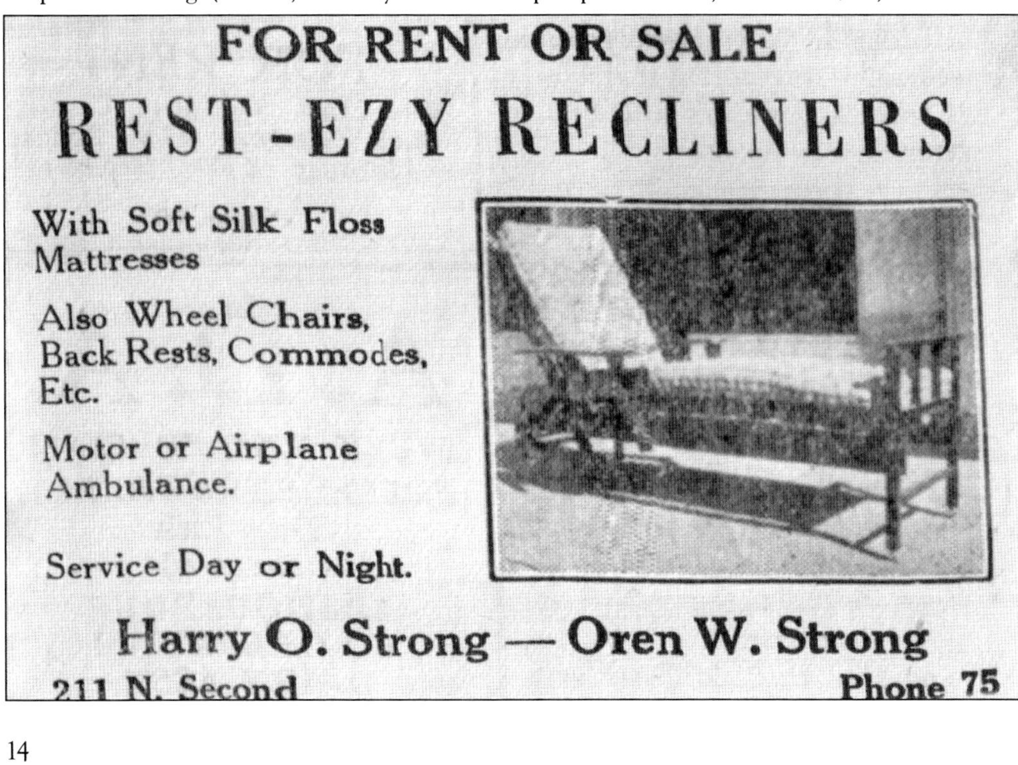

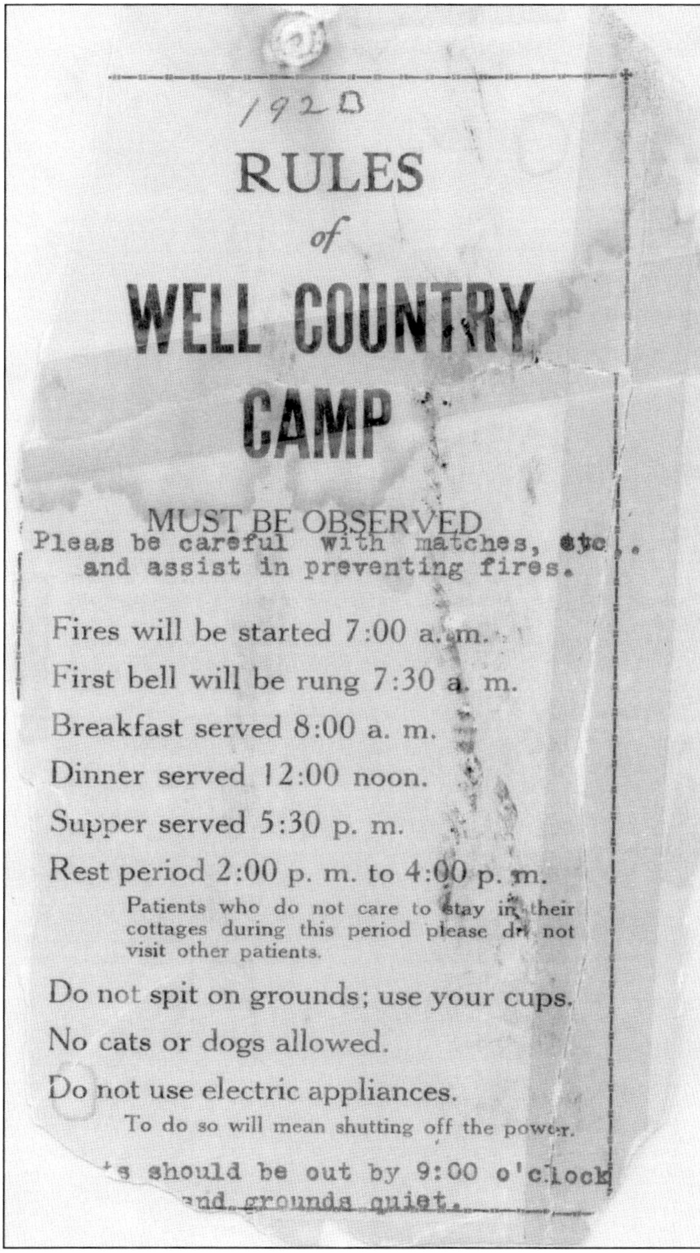

1920

RULES
of
WELL COUNTRY
CAMP
MUST BE OBSERVED

Pleas be careful with matches, etc.
and assist in preventing fires.

Fires will be started 7:00 a. m.

First bell will be rung 7:30 a. m.

Breakfast served 8:00 a. m.

Dinner served 12:00 noon.

Supper served 5:30 p. m.

Rest period 2:00 p. m. to 4:00 p. m.
Patients who do not care to stay in their cottages during this period please do not visit other patients.

Do not spit on grounds; use your cups.

No cats or dogs allowed.

Do not use electric appliances.
To do so will mean shutting off the power.

...s should be out by 9:00 o'clock
...and grounds quiet.

As important as climate, clean air, and altitude were to a lunger's recovery, more and more doctors recognized the importance of a strictly kept, regular schedule in the recovery process. Designating exact times of the day when everything should be done, sans printed schedules that included drinking hot water (7:00 a.m.), eating meals (8:00 a.m., 12:30 p.m., and 5:30 p.m.), taking temperatures and pulses (10:00 a.m., 3:00 p.m., 8:00 p.m.), and, most important, "chasing" or resting (preferably outdoors) (9:00–10:00 a.m., 11:15 a.m.–12:15 p.m., 1:00–3:00 p.m., 4:15–5:15 p.m., and 6:00–8:00 p.m.). Even resorts, like the Well Country Camp in the Sandia Mountains, distributed printed schedules, adding that "patients who do not care to stay in their cottages during [rest] period should not visit other patients" during this important time of the day. (Courtesy of Penny Hobbie.)

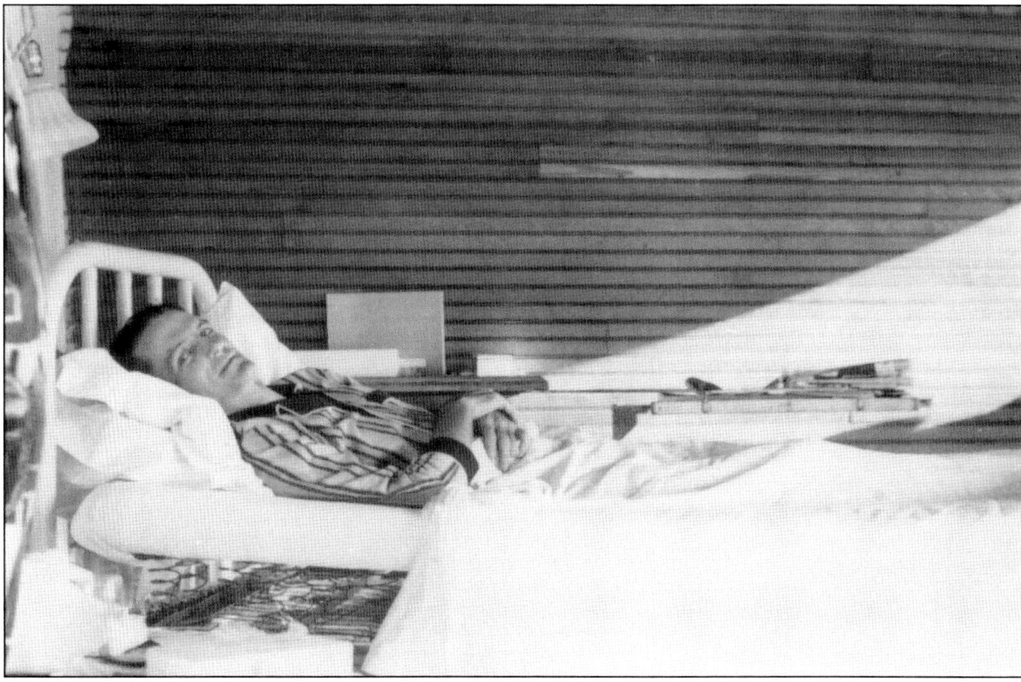

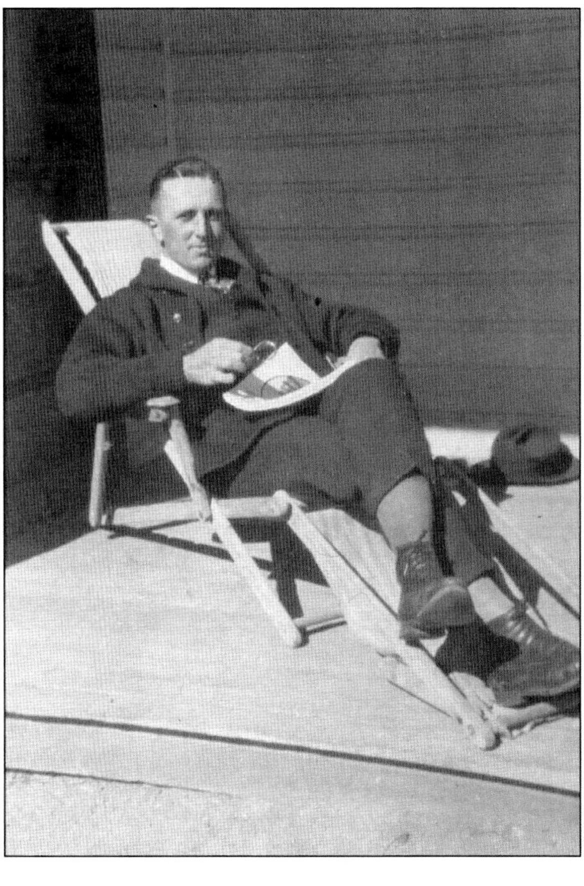

The balance of each day was given to whatever light activity a patient was well enough to attempt. Many patients "chased" diligently, especially when they first arrived, although keeping to such a tedious timetable took discipline and dedication that few people could maintain. It took semi-dictatorial doctors and nurses, who enforced schedules and kept exacting patient charts, to maintain such a rigid regimen. Adhering to such a schedule on one's own was exceedingly difficult, especially for the average young lunger living alone in New Mexico's otherwise relaxed environment. Reading, the lungers' main pastime, helped patients distract themselves for many hours. Anne Ellis's *Sunshine Preferred* (1934), which recalled her experiences at Albuquerque's Methodist san, received excellent reviews among lungers in New Mexico. (Above, courtesy of Special Collections, UNM Health Sciences Library; left, courtesy of Presbyterian Healthcare Services.)

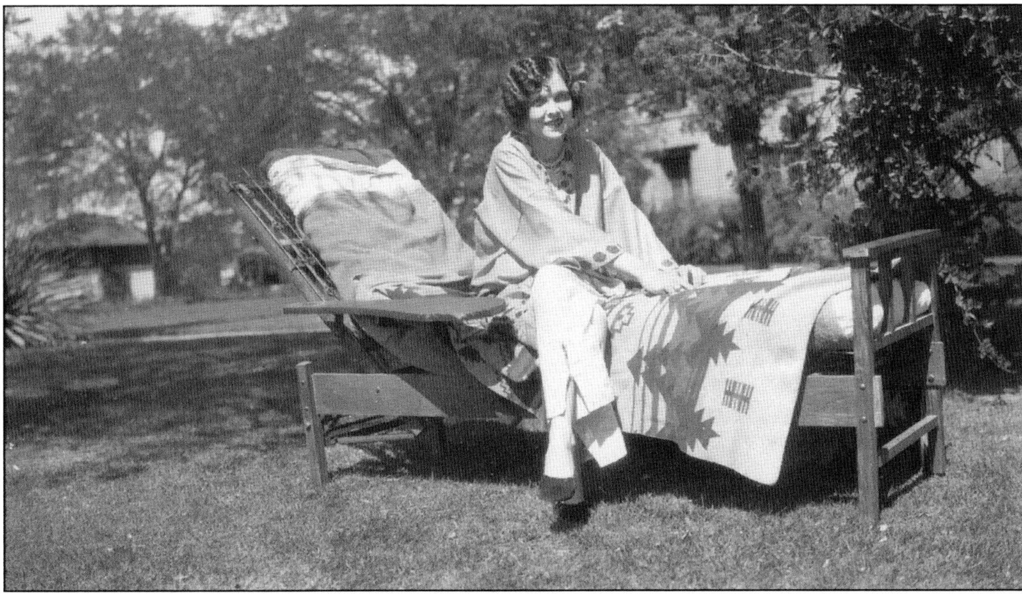

Health-seekers spent much of their day wearing pajamas, robes, and slippers. Wearing attractive bedclothes was often as essential to a lunger's self-esteem as wearing appealing street clothes had been in their previously healthy lives. Some patients outdid all others. Viola Harris at Albuquerque's Methodist Deaconess Sanatorium had so many beautiful pajamas that she became known as her san's "pajama girl" in 1930. Helen Harger won a contest for the most attractive pajamas at Albuquerque's Hillcrest san. Lungers were said to wear their best Sunday go-to-meeting pajamas on special occasions. Dress stores catered to health-seeker needs with advertisements, including for silk lounging pajamas or, as shown at right, a more practical "Curly Snuggie" with "cleverly inserted" pockets. (Above, courtesy of the Albuquerque Museum, PA1982.181.432.)

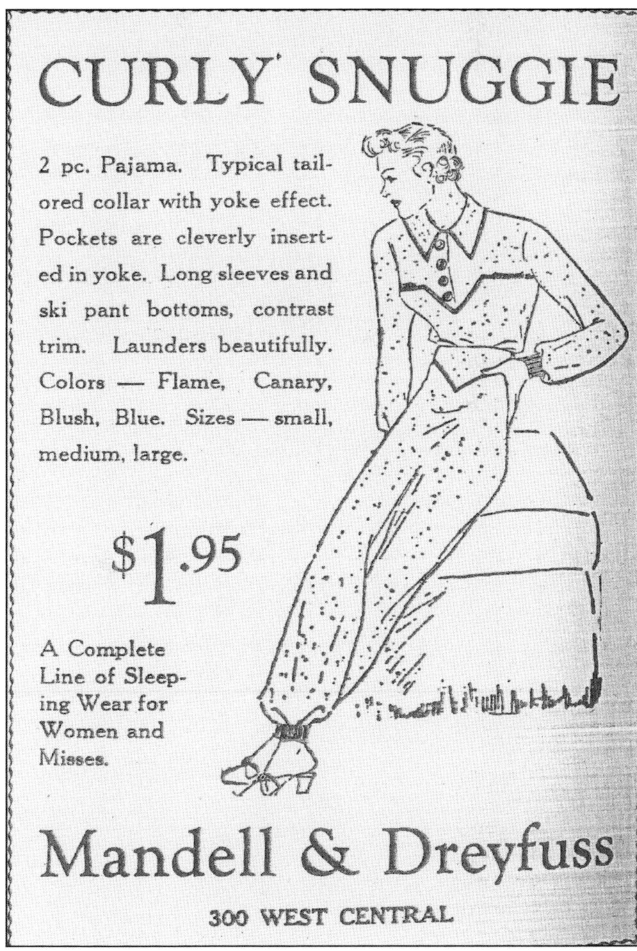

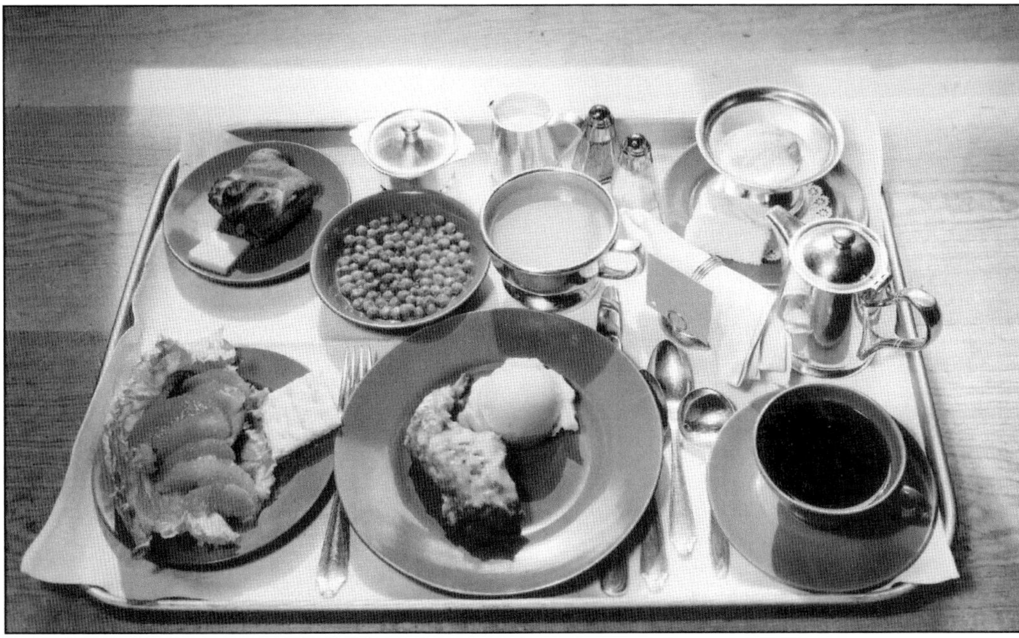

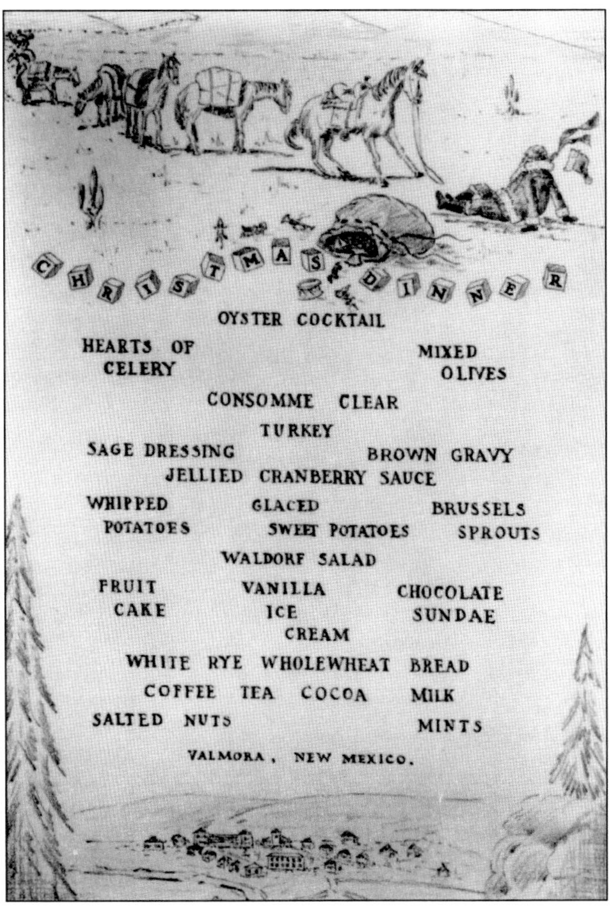

Hyperalimentation (eating to compensate for excessive weight loss) was considered an essential part of a lunger's recovery. Patients were weighed regularly to measure weight gains—or losses. Patients ate as often as six times a day, with dieticians including as many as two-dozen raw eggs and four quarts of milk in a patient's daily menu. Patients at the Fort Stanton Marine Hospital consumed as much as 4,026 calories a day; the average active male requires no more than 3,000. A doctor at St. Joseph recalled, "All we did for TB [patients] was put them to bed, gave them fresh air, and [administer] *forced feedings.*" Weight gains were big news, as when Earl Johnson at Albuquerque's Methodist san gained 10 pounds in 11 days in 1938. (Above, courtesy of Presbyterian Healthcare Services; left, courtesy of Special Collections, UNM Health Sciences Library.)

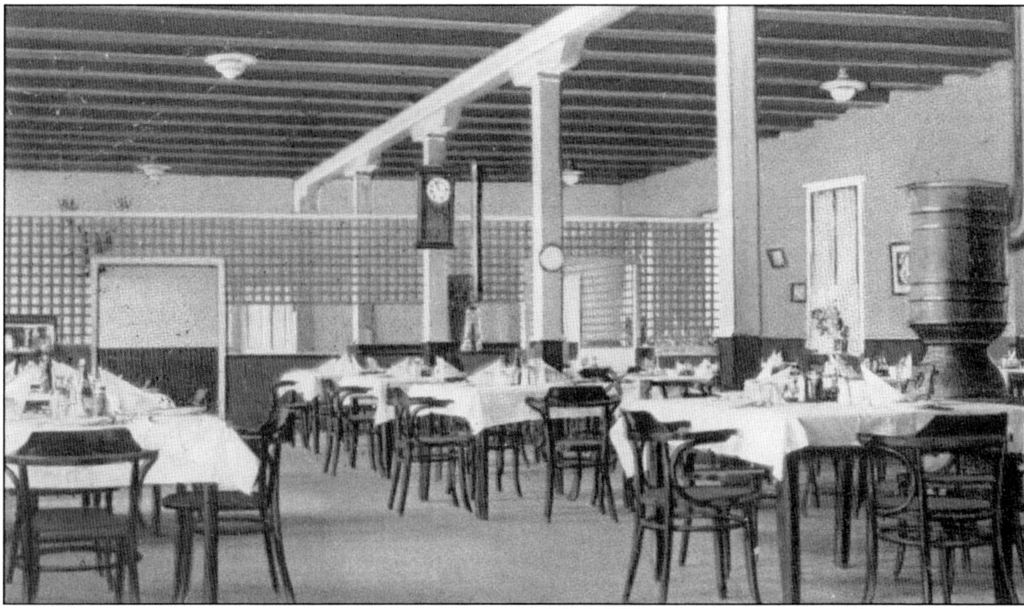

Access to a san's dining room was considered a major step in a patient's recovery. When Grace Edmister took her first meal with other patients at Albuquerque's St. Joseph san, they drank champagne to celebrate the occasion. In 1928, John Ransom at the Valmora Sanatorium sent this postcard to his mother, writing, "This is where I went to eat for the first time last nite. The X is about where I sit."

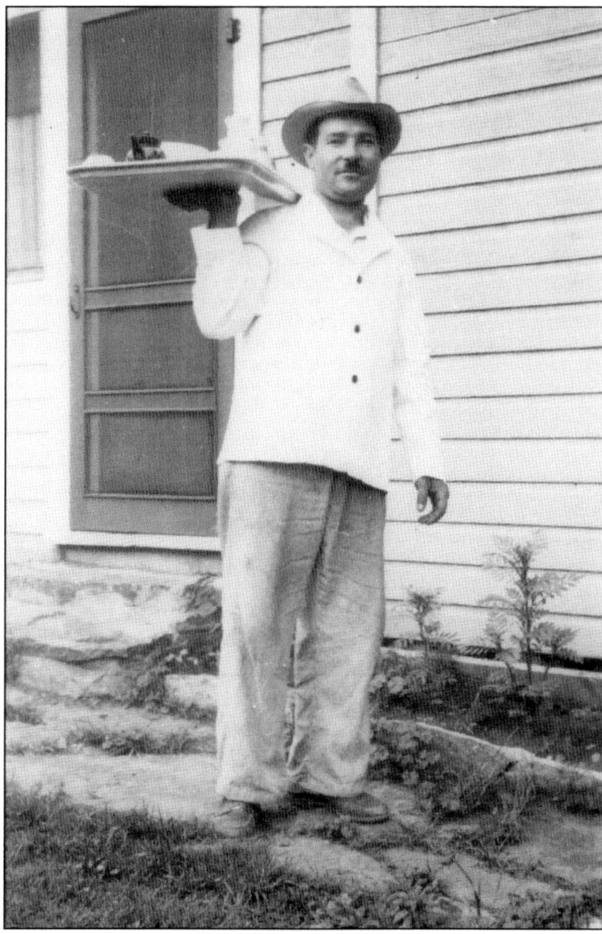

If not ready for meals in the dining room, patients remained in their rooms, where "tray boys" (and at least two "tray girls") delivered their meals. These employees raced with trays balanced on their shoulders to make sure that hot meals were delivered hot. Eager to amuse patients, some tray boys performed clever stunts, including dance steps while miraculously balancing their trays. (Courtesy of Special Collections, UNM Health Sciences Library.)

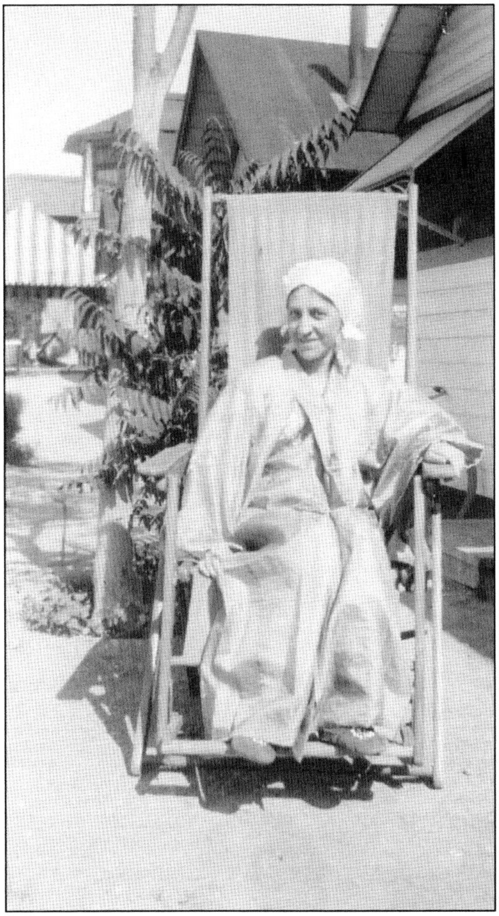

Abundant fresh air, food, and rest were essential elements in a patient like Nellie Weigand's recovery, but so was a positive attitude. Paul Doran recalls Dr. Carl Mulky, one of New Mexico's best-known TB specialists, telling him that Albuquerque's cemeteries were full of lungers with less TB than Paul had, because they had succumbed to a poor attitude about their chances of recovery. Mulky said that TB killed a patient in the head, not in the lungs. Doran asserted that a sense of humor was especially valuable in avoiding depression, or what was commonly known as a "TB personality." (Both, courtesy of Presbyterian Healthcare Services.)

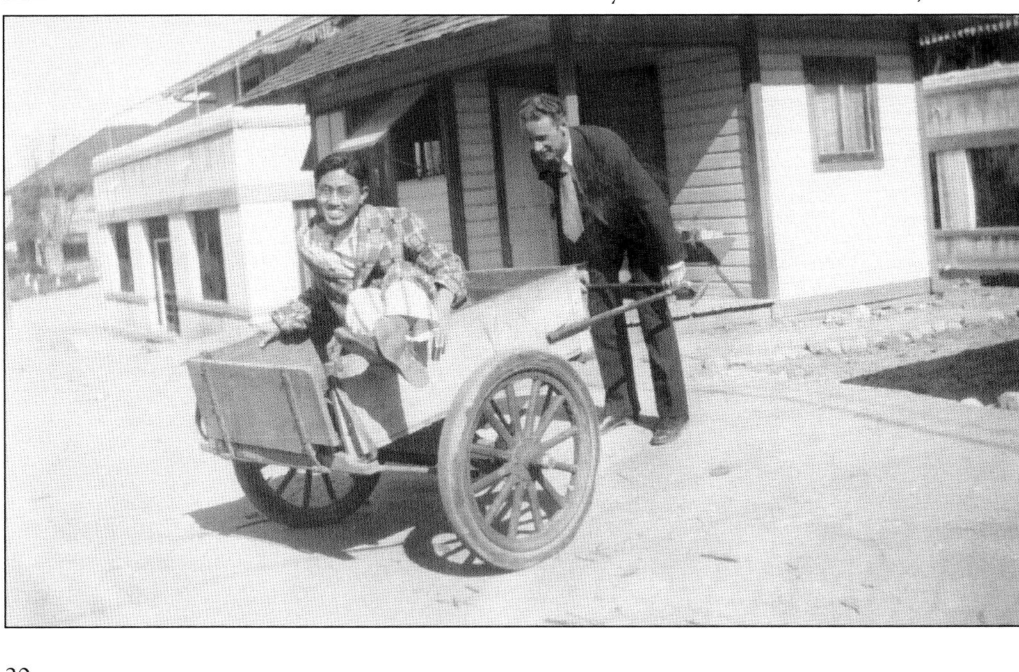

Two

Santa Fe's St. Vincent and Sunmount Sanatoriums

With its fine weather, high altitude, and railroad connections (or at least a spur line from Lamy, New Mexico), Santa Fe, the *Santa Fe New Mexican* declared, had become the "world's sanitarium" by 1892. Eager to promote its health-seeker advantages, the *New Mexican* ran an identical article nearly every day in 1899 and 1900. Its headlines trumpeted Santa Fe's "Superb Climate" and "Fine Summers and Moderate Winters." A temperature table favorably compared Santa Fe's temperature to cities like Chicago and New York. Nearly everyone in Santa Fe agreed with the *New Mexican's* desire to attract "a well-to-do class of health seekers and tourists" who could be expected to "expend vast sums of money." The smallest interest in establishing a new san stirred excitement and produced front-page headlines in the capital.

Santa Fe would host two of New Mexico's most famous, longest-lasting sans—St. Vincent's and Sunmount. Other, smaller facilities included the high-end Diaz Sanitarium, the Charles F. Lummis Sanatorium (now the Santa Fe Indian Hospital), and even a five-bed ward for tubercular inmates at the state penitentiary.

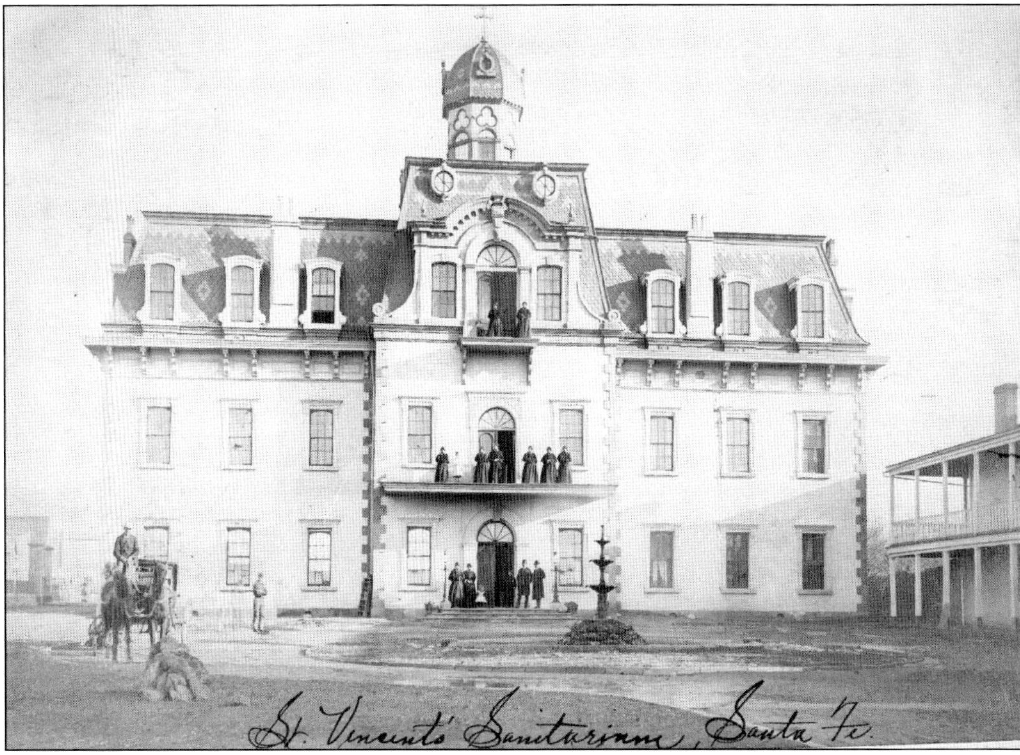

Four members of the Sisters of Charity from Cincinnati, Ohio, arrived in Santa Fe by coach on June 15, 1865. Invited to New Mexico by the territory's first bishop, Jean Baptiste Lamy, the sisters opened a temporary hospital, named St. Vincent's, in part of the bishop's residency. The hospital was the first of its kind in the territory and a major part of Lamy's grand plans to bring Catholic social institutions, including schools, orphanages, and hospitals, to the Southwest. The hospital accommodated patients with various ailments, of which TB was most prevalent. (Both, courtesy of the Museum of New Mexico—above, no. 67744, below, no. 61376.)

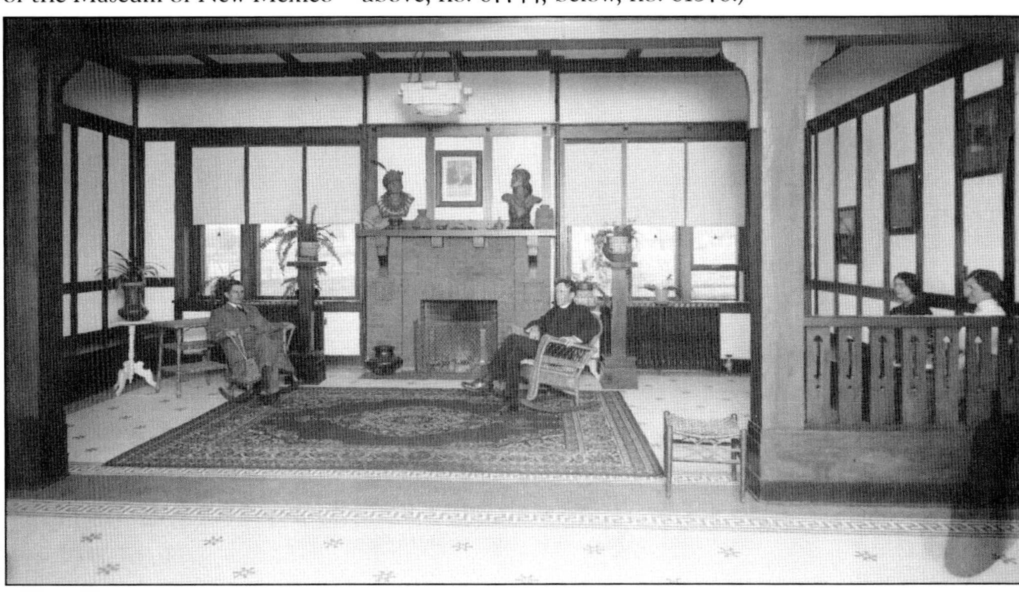

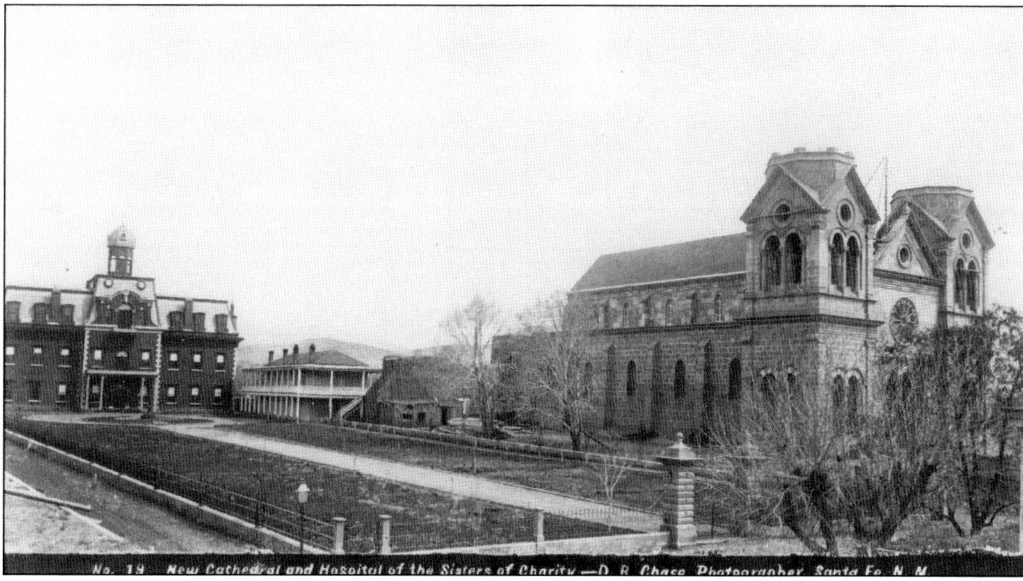
No. 19 New Cathedral and Hospital of the Sisters of Charity—D. B. Chase Photographer, Santa Fe, N. M.

St. Vincent's began to attract health-seekers from across the country. With so many new patients, a three-story building that had been erected as an industrial school for girls instead became a sanatorium. It was the tallest building in Santa Fe. Unfortunately, Santa Fe's first san burned down in a fire on June 14, 1896. The Sisters of Charity rescued 56 patients in their hospital and san. Although the bells at St. Francis Cathedral sounded the alarm, and local firemen responded quickly, poor firefighting equipment and a lack of water pressure hampered efforts to extinguish the flames. Local fireman John Fayette was badly injured. The blaze, of unknown origin, caused up to $75,000 in damages. Tragically, most of the hospital's insurance had recently expired. (Above, courtesy of the Museum of New Mexico, no. 15167.)

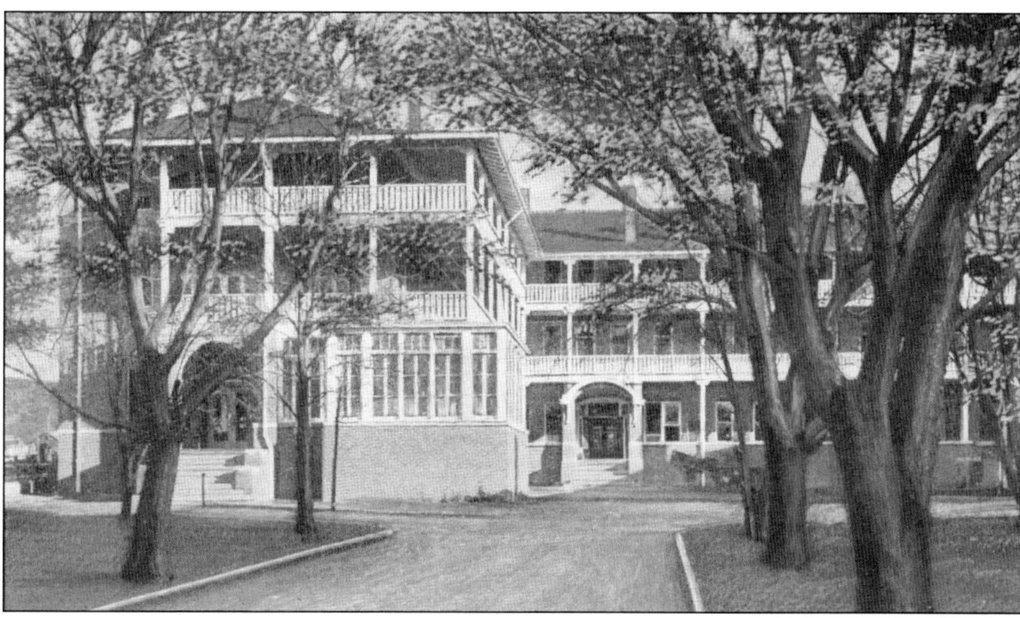

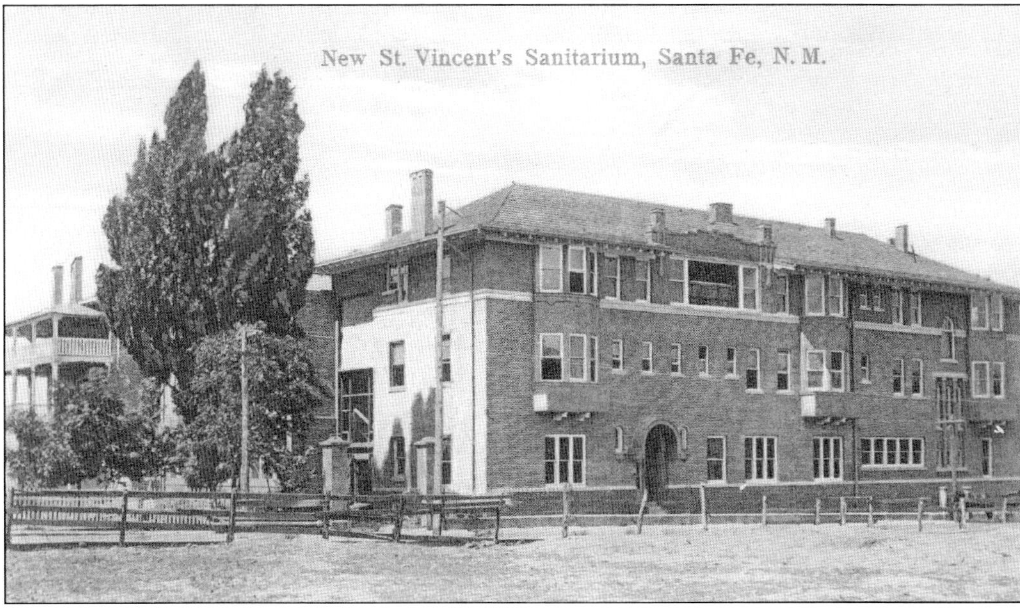

Despite the san's 1896 fire, St. Vincent's rebuilt and continued to receive new patients. In 1900, thirty-six lungers received care, with applications for rooms arriving almost daily. A larger san was finally built and opened on December 14, 1910. The *Santa Fe New Mexican* praised the new facility's modern kitchen, hot and cold running water in each patient's room, 75 beds, 4 suites, electric call buttons, and comfortable sleeping porches. A modern elevator was installed, although it often failed to work, meaning that doctors and nurses sometimes had to carry patients to their rooms on upper floors. (Below, courtesy of the Museum of New Mexico, no. 61372.)

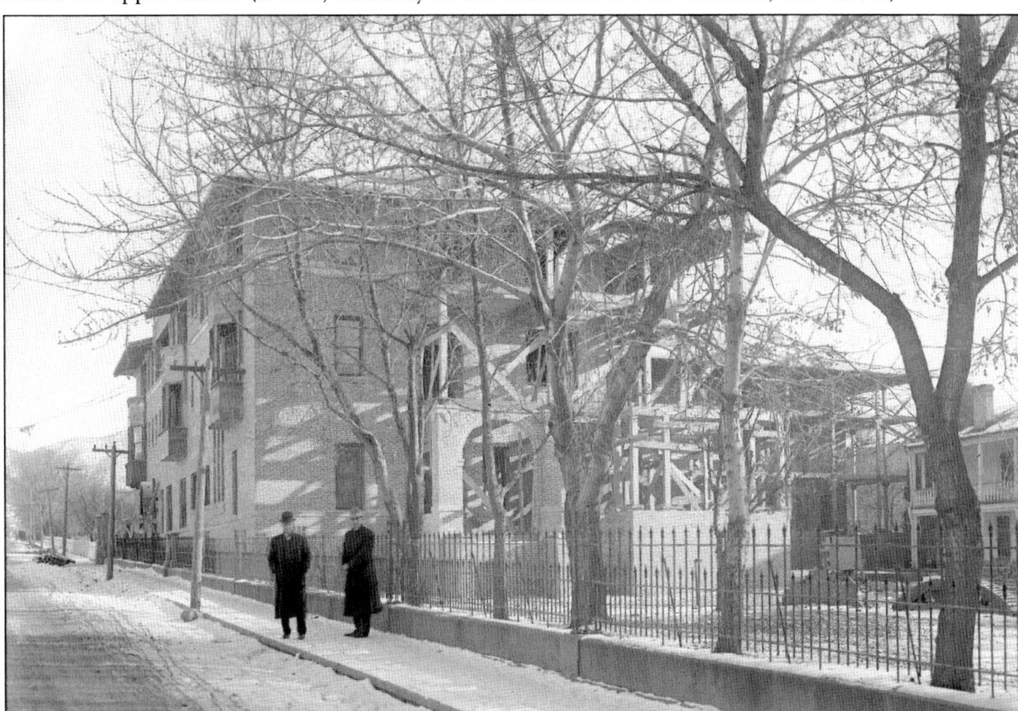

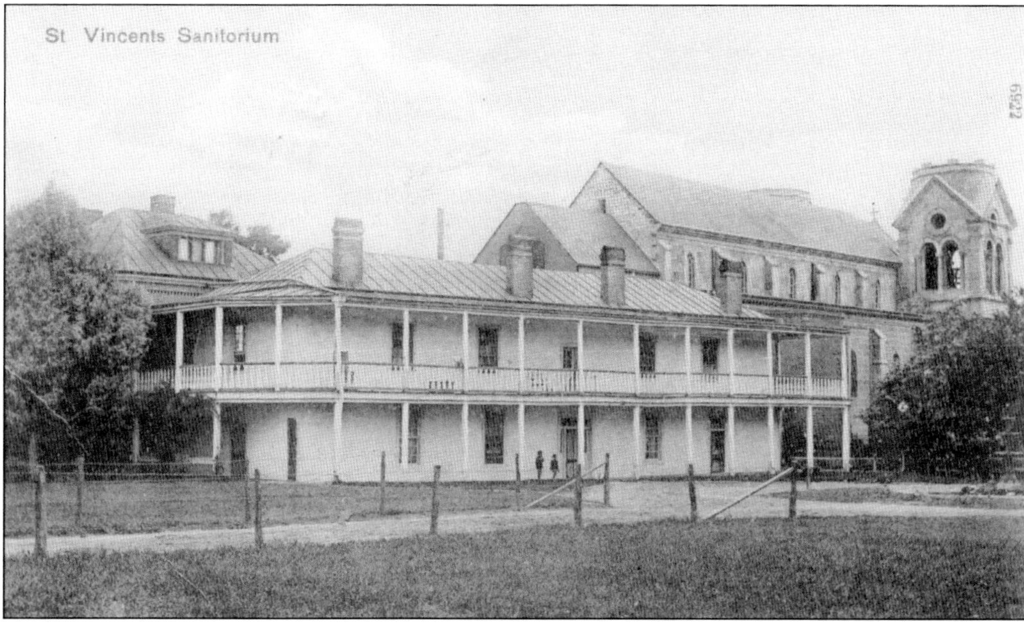

The new, safer sanatorium and hospital functioned well for four decades. Many patients were cared for, with hundreds recovering, although others died of TB and other illnesses. Nearby St. Francis Cathedral rang its bells whenever someone died at St. Vincent's, until patients at the san complained, saying that the tolling bells had an adverse impact on their mental health and physical recovery. (Courtesy of Jim Coad.)

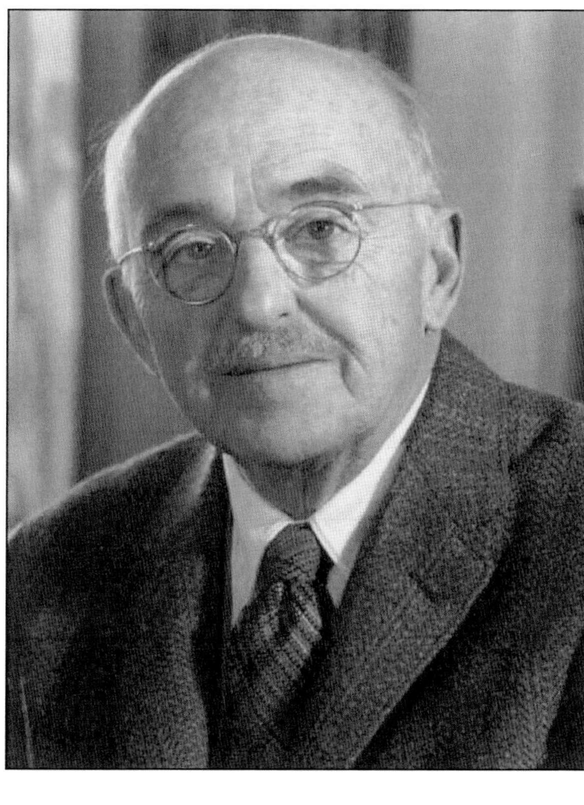

By 1950, the hospital that had seemed so modern in 1910 had become obsolete. A new St. Vincent's, designed by former lunger John Gaw Meem (pictured), opened in 1953. When St. Vincent's moved to St. Michael's Drive in 1977, the building on East Palace Avenue became a nursing home. Reportedly haunted, the property was sold in 2007, with plans to make it into a luxury hotel.

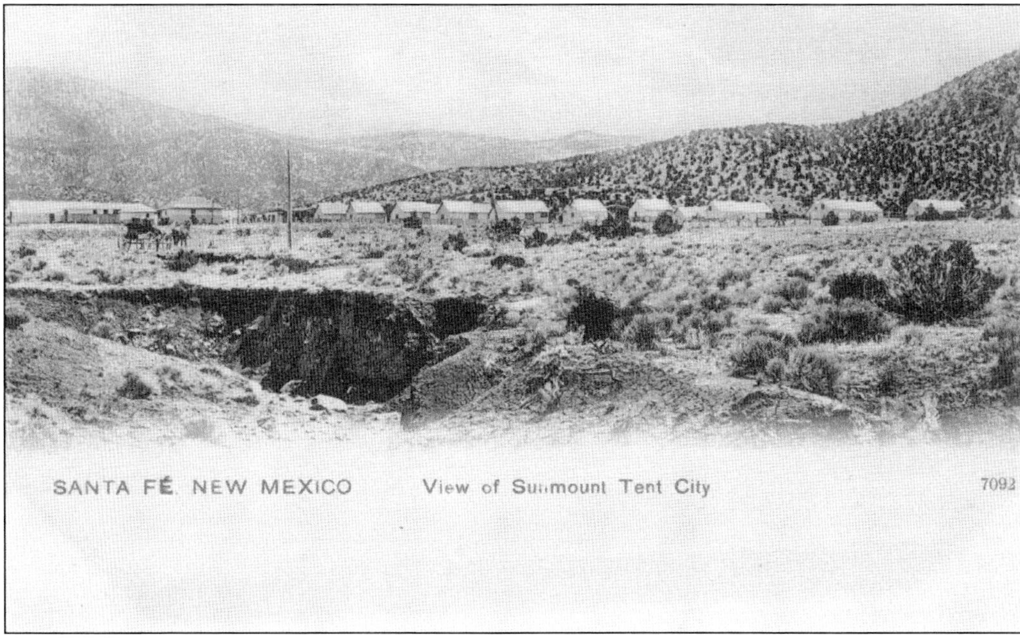
SANTA FÉ. NEW MEXICO
View of Sunmount Tent City
7092

Opened by Mayor A.R. Gibson and F.H. Mitchell in November 1903, Santa Fe's Sunmount Tent City (above) was hailed in the *Santa Fe New Mexican* as a health mecca with prices "within the reach of all," a clear advantage over expensive sanatoriums elsewhere in the Southwest. Modeled after San Diego's Coronado Tent City, Sunmount included about three dozen tents, each with an iron bed, a mattress, bed clothing, carpet, and a stove. Costs ranged from $7 to $10 a month. Meals were an extra $5 per week. A main building (below) housed administrative offices, a dining room, and an entertainment hall. The san offered pure water (from nearby mountain springs), a phone line to Santa Fe, horse stables, poultry for eggs, and Jersey cows for milk. (Above, courtesy of Jim Coad; below, courtesy of the Immaculate Heart of Mary Retreat Conference Center.)

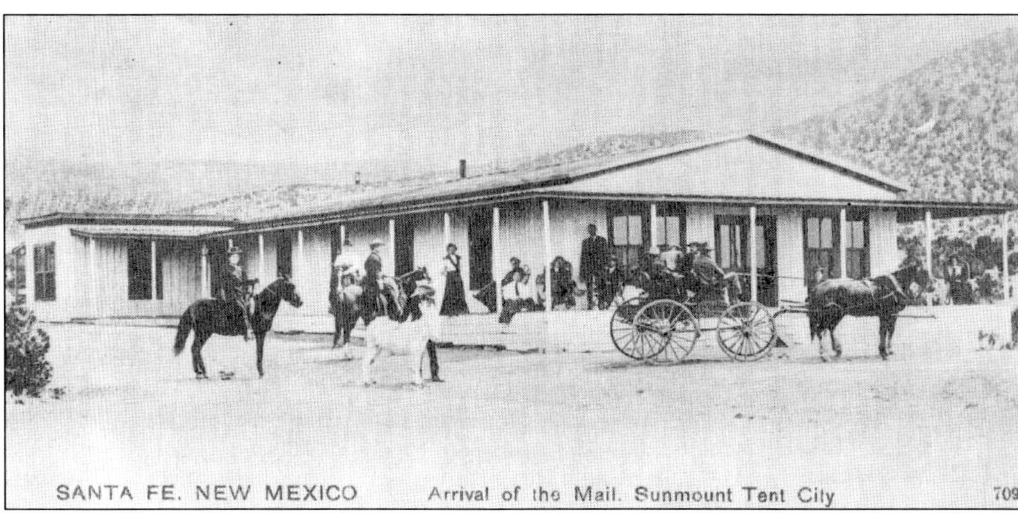
SANTA FE. NEW MEXICO
Arrival of the Mail. Sunmount Tent City
7091

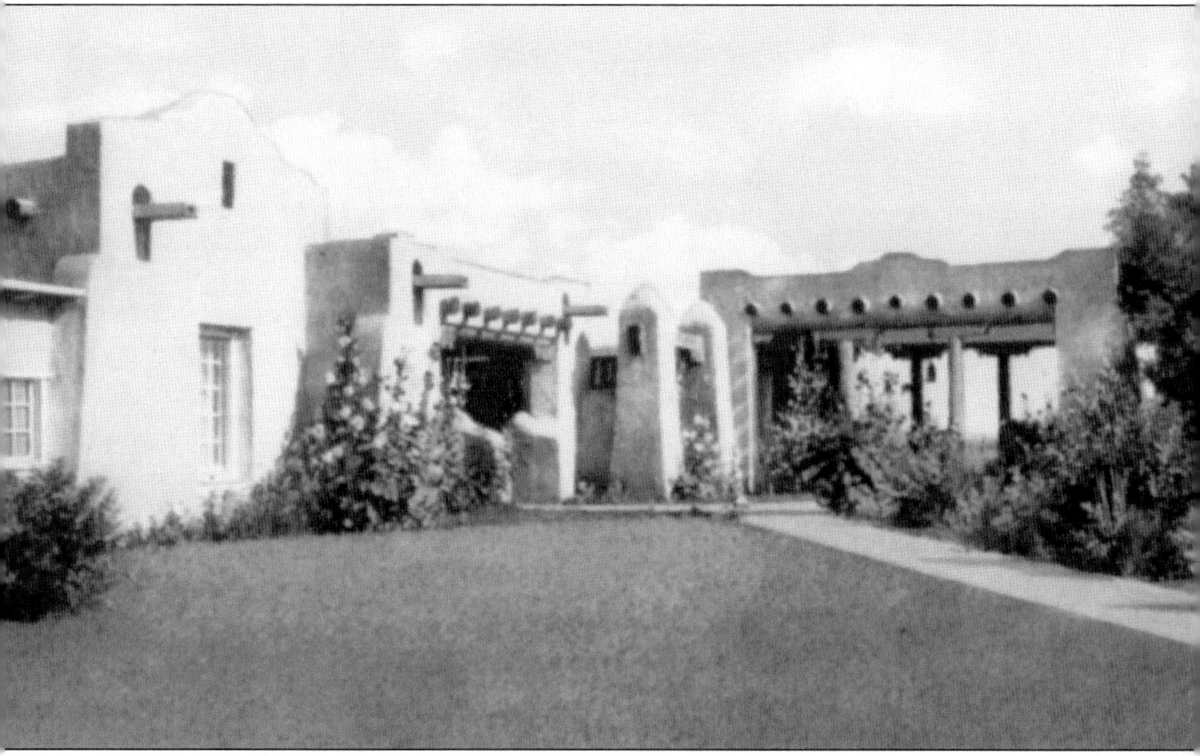

Located a mile and a half south of the Santa Fe Plaza, at the corner of Camino del Monte Sol and the Old Santa Fe Trail, the Sunmount Tent Colony in reality offered little beyond high elevation, fresh air, and proximity to town. Dr. Frank E. Mera and his brother Dr. Harry P. Mera Jr. were well aware of these shortcomings when they purchased the tent colony in 1906. Frank was a health-seeker who had just spent two years recovering from TB in a Colorado Springs san. Eager to open a san to institute his own ideas, he began to replace tents with cottages designed to encourage rest in a relaxed setting, the antithesis of impersonal, institutional hospital rooms. In 1914, Frank commissioned Isaac Rapp to design the san's first Pueblo Revival–style buildings, which, according to architectural historian Chris Wilson, symbolized "a harmonious Pueblo village far from the tensions of urban industrial life."

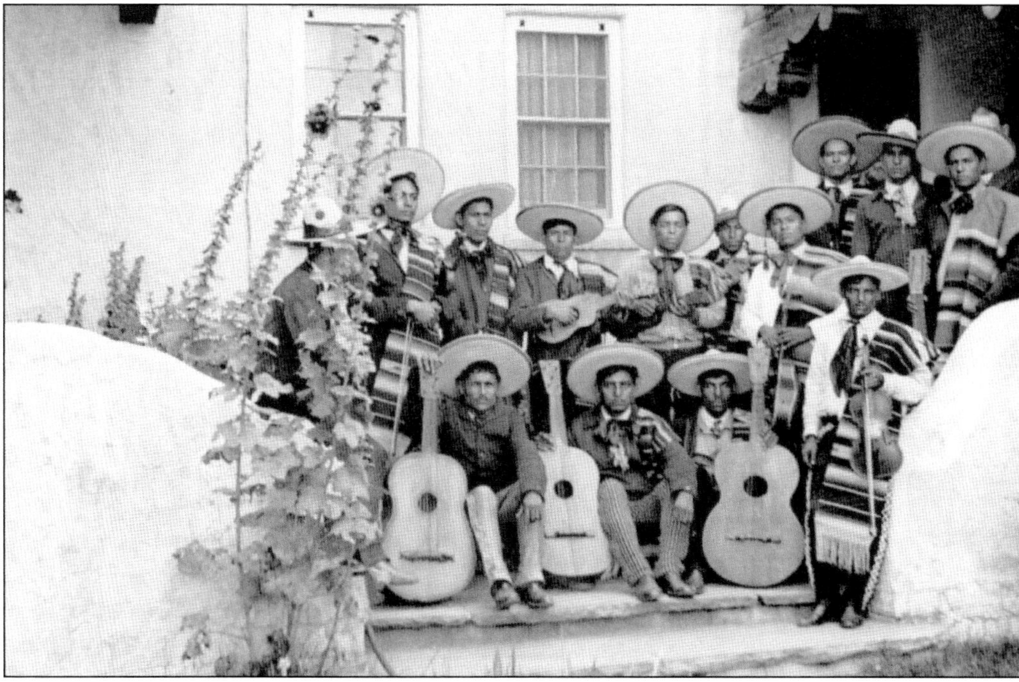

Frank Mera hoped to attract lungers to his new san by creating an intellectually stimulating environment conducive to both emotional and physical healing. Mera recruited such talented poets and authors as Mary Austin, Carl Sandburg, and Witter Bynner to read from their works and discuss their meaning at weekly salons. Sylvanus G. Morley and Edgar Lee Hewitt shared their anthropological findings. Artists and musicians, including mariachis, were invited as well. In a typical presentation in 1926, mask maker Howard Coluzzi appeared at an informal tea to describe the fashions of masks in history. Sunmount became a natural extension of the growing Santa Fe art colony. Santa Fe's intellectual environment proved nearly as invigorating as its salubrious climate. (Both, courtesy of the John Gaw Meem Collection, New Mexico State Records Center and Archives.)

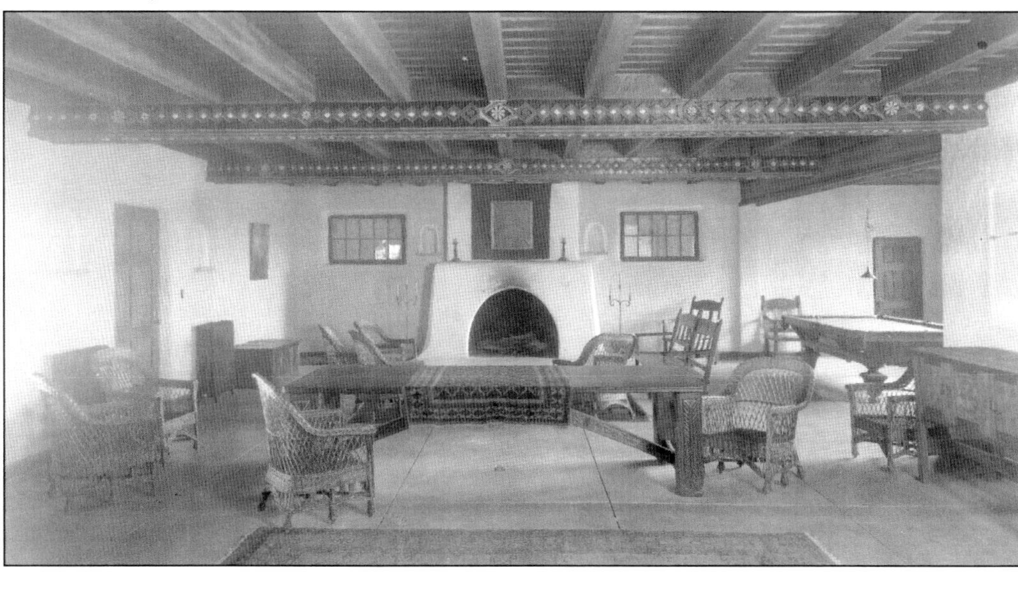

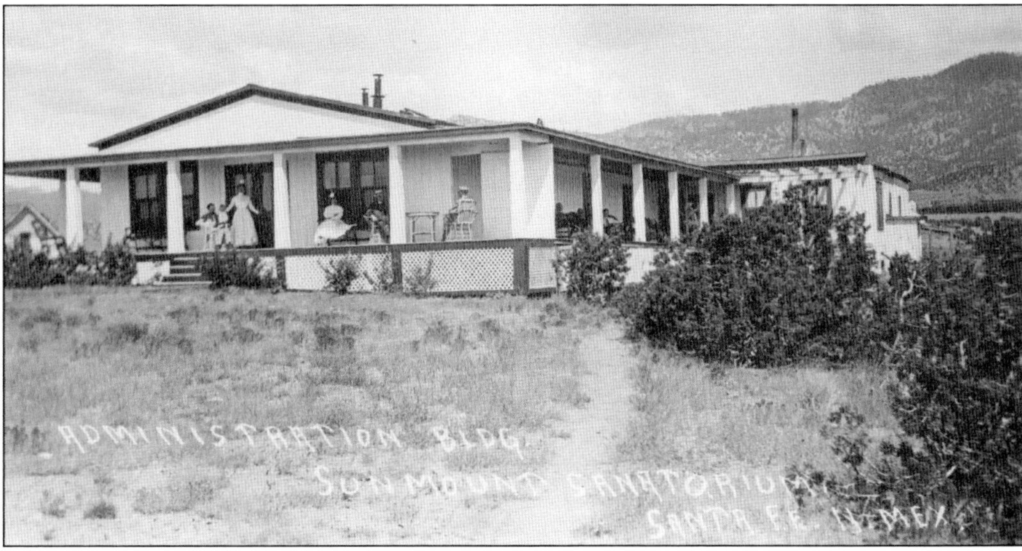

Sunmount's comfortable cottages included sleeping porches with views of the nearby Sangre de Cristo Mountains. One wonders if Harry Mera, an archaeologist who used the Zia symbol to design the New Mexico state flag, was hoping to create a place for healing that reflected the Zia Pueblo's four sacred obligations—development of a strong body, a clear mind, a pure spirit, and devotion to the care of others. Strong friendships and romantic relationships inevitably developed in such an environment. Katherine Stinson, known as the "School Girl Flyer" during her exciting aviation career, was diagnosed with TB in 1918. While recovering at Sunmount, she met Miguel Otero, a fellow lunger and the son of a former territorial governor. The couple married in 1927 and enjoyed a happy 50-year marriage. (Both, courtesy of the Museum of New Mexico—above, no. 23089, below, no. 61398.)

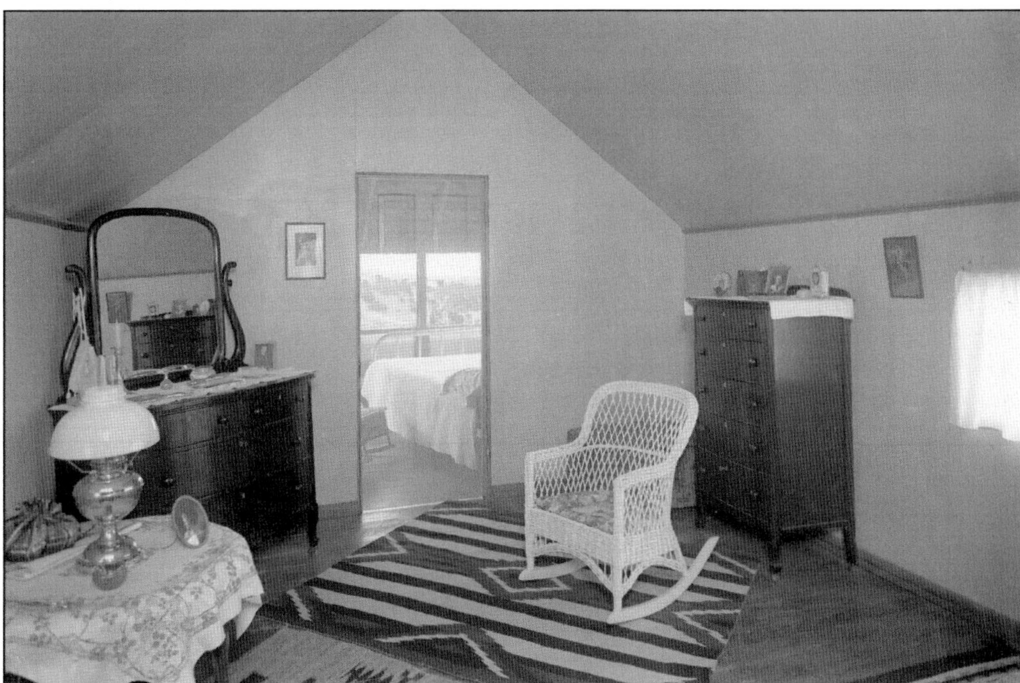

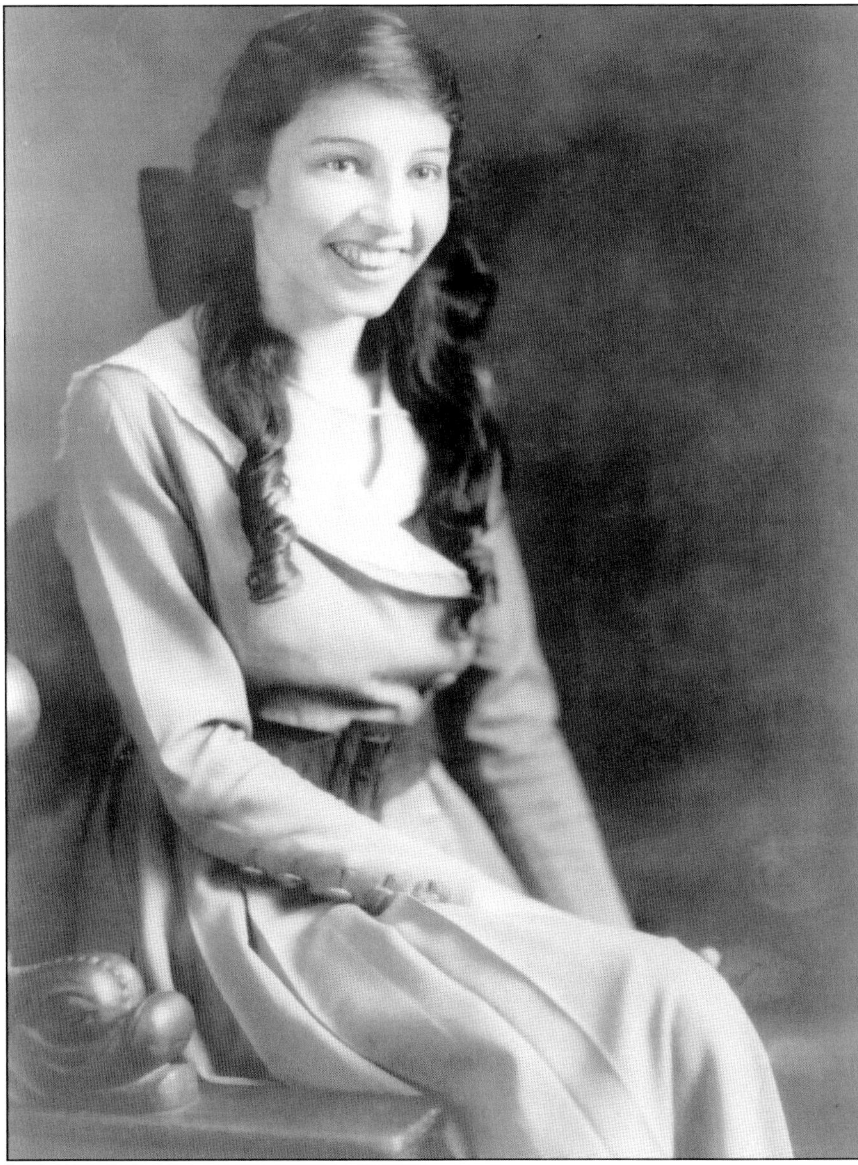

Frank Mera created a congenial, creative community where many lungers developed their nascent talents or discovered entirely new ones. Arriving in 1916, twenty-year-old Alice Corbin Henderson soon blossomed as a poet and social leader. Lynn Riggs found increasing self-confidence as a young author and poet. Dr. Robert O. Brown recovered to become the medical director at St. Vincent's and one of the most respected TB experts in the Southwest. Katherine Stinson-Otero (shown here) discovered an interest in Southwest architecture and devoted much of her 86-year life to her new profession. Her husband, lunger Miguel Otero, became a respected judge. Dorothy McKibbin recovered to play a key role as the "gatekeeper" to Los Alamos during World War II. John Gaw Meem arrived at Sunmount as a young engineer, leaving the san 18 months later to become the foremost advocate of Southwest architecture in New Mexico history. Appropriately, he was a chief architect in the building or remodeling of the Bataan Memorial Methodist Hospital (formerly the Methodist Deaconess Sanatorium), St. Vincent's in Santa Fe, and Presbyterian in Albuquerque.

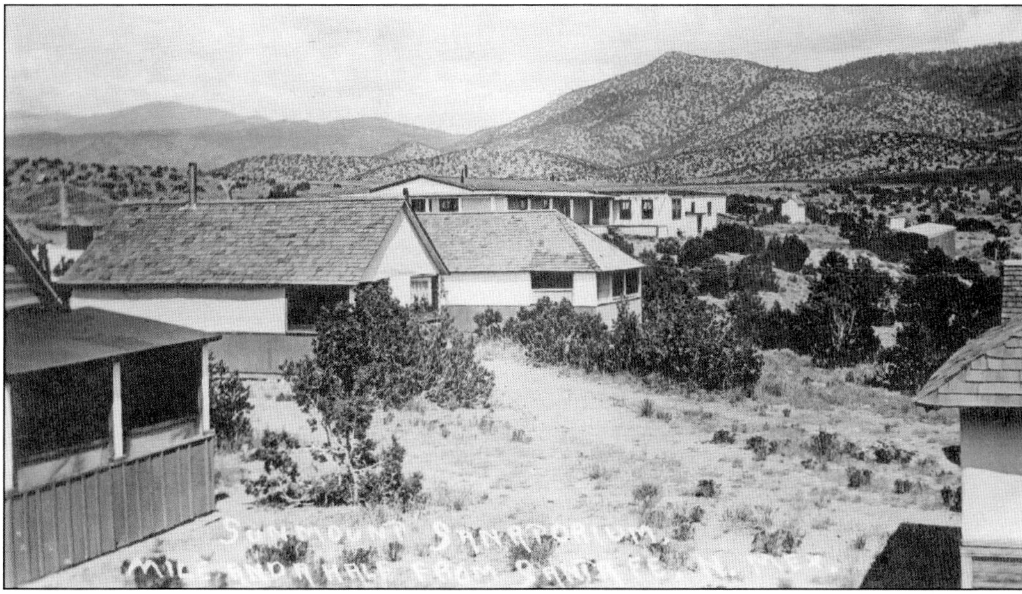

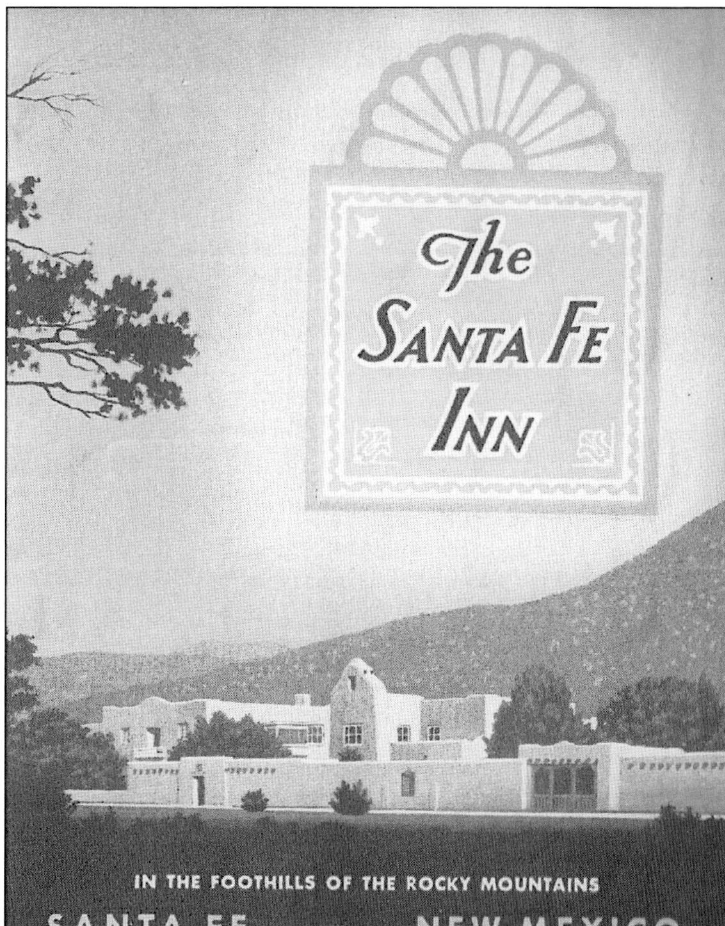

Frank Mera owned and operated Sunmount for nearly 40 years. His san enjoyed a high rate of success among lungers, based not only on its unique environment, but also on the fact that Mera only admitted patients in the early stages of TB. With fewer lungers arriving in Santa Fe by 1937, Mera announced that he hoped to remodel the san to make it a resort hotel, to be called the Santa Fe Inn. The inn failed to develop, leaving Mera to sell the property to the Catholic Church. (Above, courtesy of Jim Coad; right, courtesy of the Immaculate Heart of Mary Retreat Conference Center.)

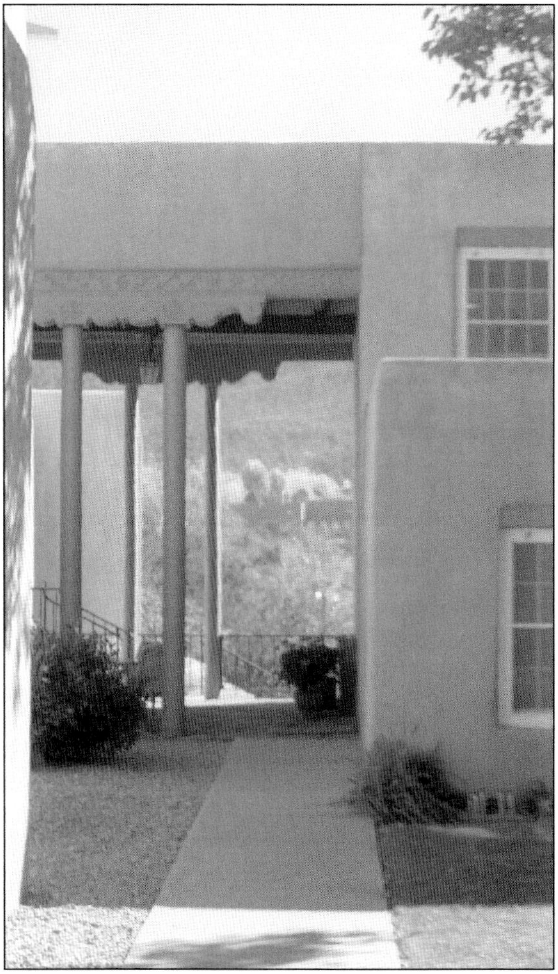

Since 1946, Sunmount has served as a monastery for the Sisters of Carmelite Order and, more recently, as the peaceful Immaculate Heart of Mary Retreat and Conference Center. The sanatorium's environment was usually just as peaceful, but there were at least some rowdy exceptions. In 1959, Santa Fe poet Witter Bynner recalled an evening at Sunmount when Dr. Mera went to a movie and the patients "dug out" some liquor, played records, and danced a new "wild, barbaric dance" called the Fibla. The evening ended on Mera's return, but, in Bynner's words, "it was real fun while it lasted and, as far as I know, no one died."

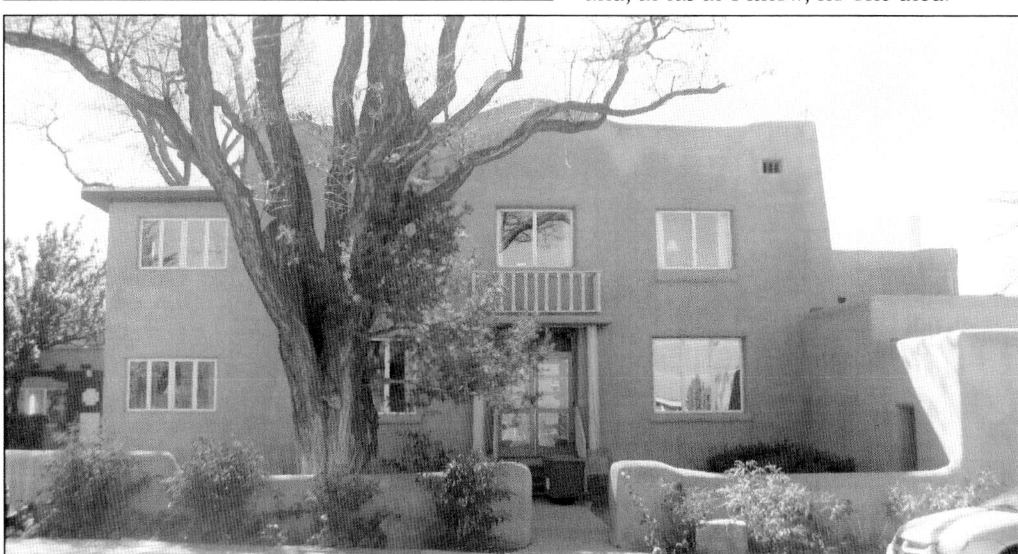

Three

Albuquerque's St. Joseph Sanatorium

The Sisters of Charity founded St. Joseph, Albuquerque's first sanatorium and hospital, on May 30, 1902. With Sister Zit Denman as its director and Dr. J.H. Wroth as its medical director, the new hospital came to specialize in the treatment of tuberculosis. Its original $50,000 building was largely financed by the sisters' motherhouse in Mount St. Joseph, Ohio, although local residents showed their support by raising $5,000 at bazaars and furnishing individual rooms, as was done by wealthy businessmen like Solomon Luna and Felipe Chavez. Because the san was about a mile from downtown Albuquerque, T.S. Hubbell gave the sisters a horse, W.L. Trimble gave them a carriage, and O.W. Strong & Sons, a mortuary, contributed an ambulance. All were optimistic about the institution and its future. None could have imagined that St. Joseph would serve as one of Albuquerque's three major health centers for the next 101 years.

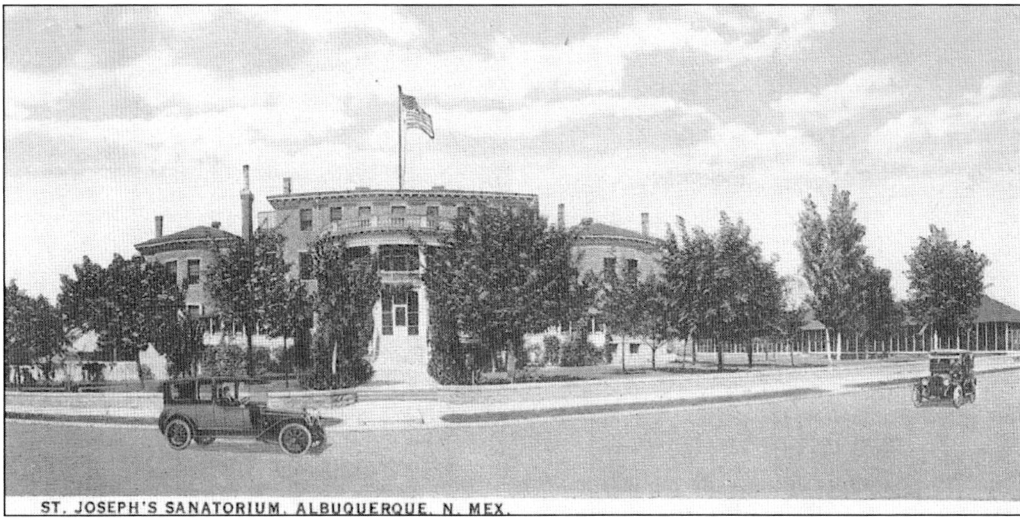

Like those at most sans, St. Joseph activities were centered in a large administration building, usually housing offices, reception rooms, a lounge, a dining room, the kitchen, and medical facilities. According to landscape historian Kristen Reynolds, these buildings functioned as "entrance points," designed to be "as impressive as money allowed" to properly welcome visiting physicians, prospective patients, worried families, and likely financial supporters in a warm, appealing setting.

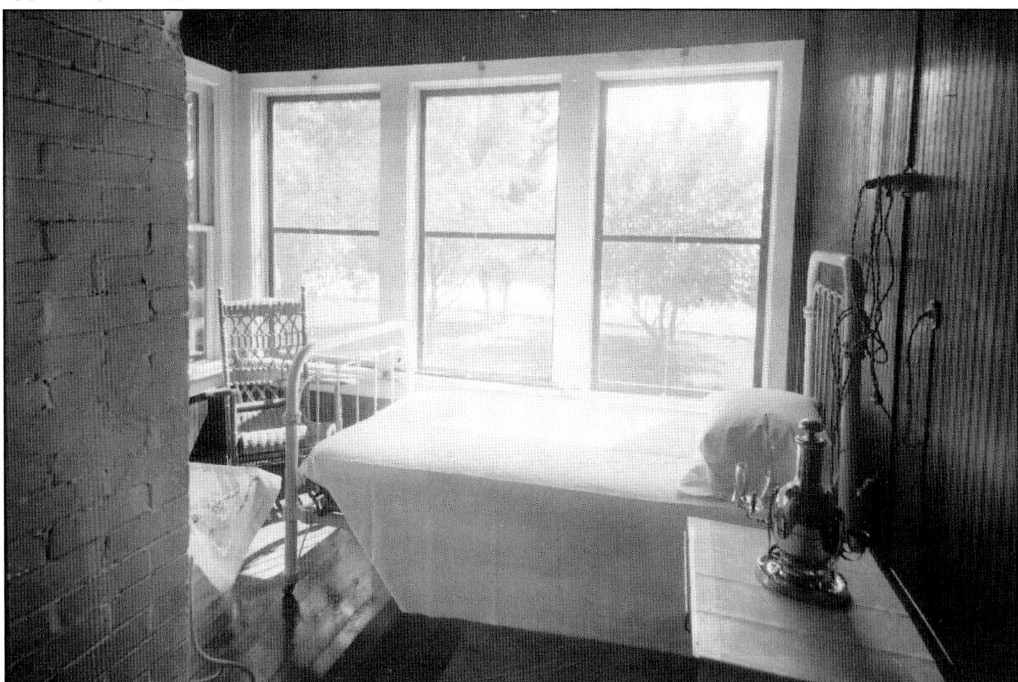

St. Joseph admitted 517 patients in its first year of operation alone. Its original building had many large windows, allowing access to plenty of fresh air, warm sunshine, and beautiful views. Rooms were designed to be as homelike as possible, making middle-class patients feel like catered-to guests, rather than like inmates in sterile institutions. (Courtesy of the Albuquerque Museum, PA1992.5.446.)

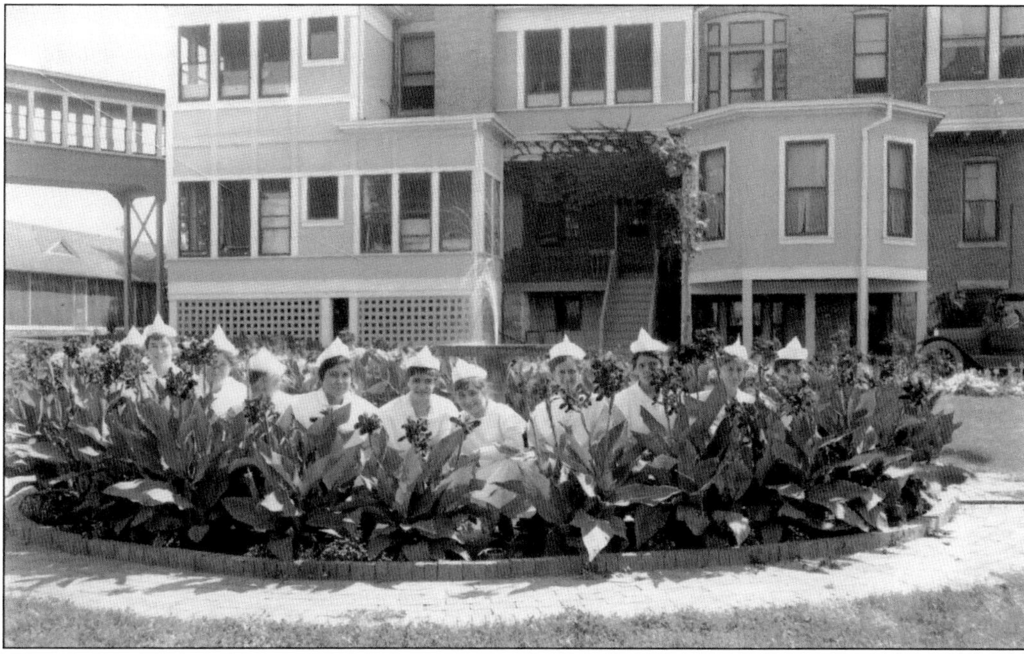

Finding that its need for trained nurses far exceeded the local supply, St. Joseph opened its own nursing school soon after the san was established. The school's first graduate, Jennie Gavin, was capped in 1905. The Regina School trained as many as 50 nurses at a time. Most students came from New Mexico; a majority were Anglo. By 1952, some 500 women had "bloomed" (graduated). (Courtesy of the Albuquerque Museum, PA1992.5.465.)

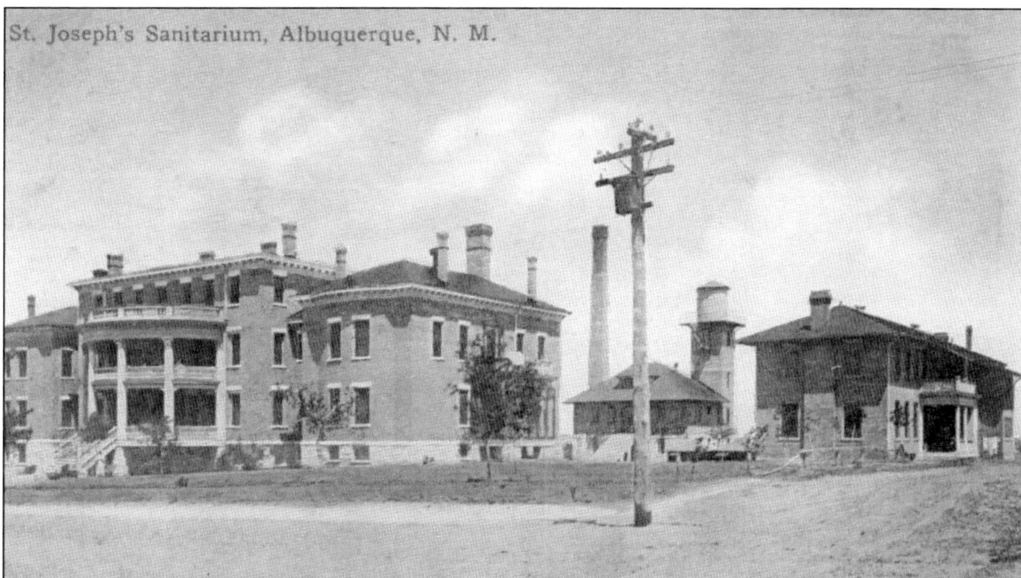

St. Joseph boasted its own heating plant, water tower, and electrical power to provide everyday utilities. The san nevertheless faced its share of crises. Lunger Irene Fisher remembered escaping through a window when a fire broke out in the san's kitchen in 1920. A decade later, when a blaze started behind the cottages, male patients formed a water-bucket brigade to dowse the flames until the local fire department arrived.

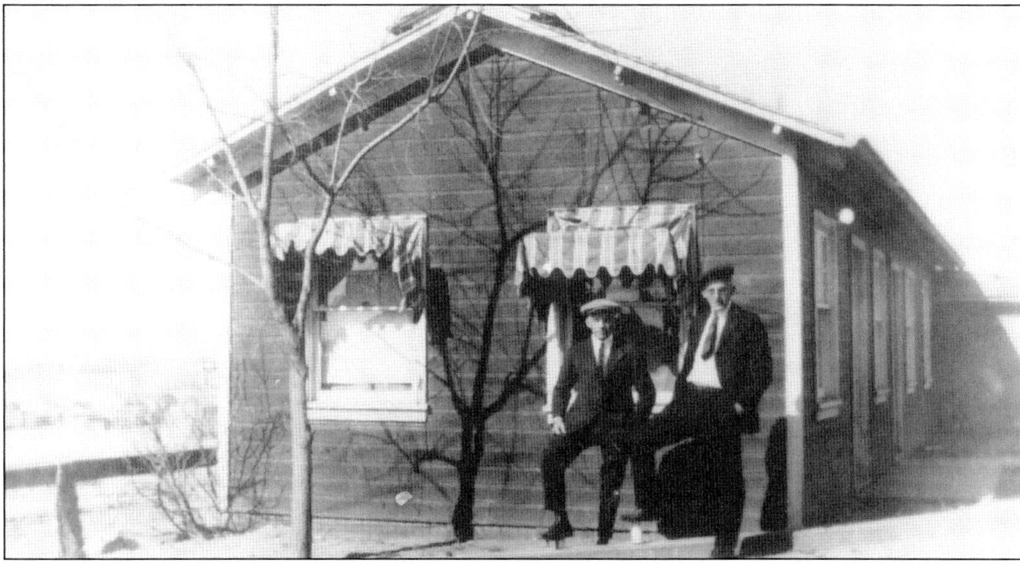

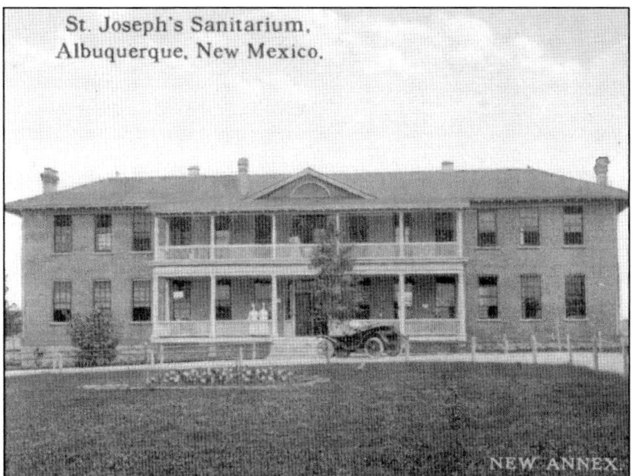

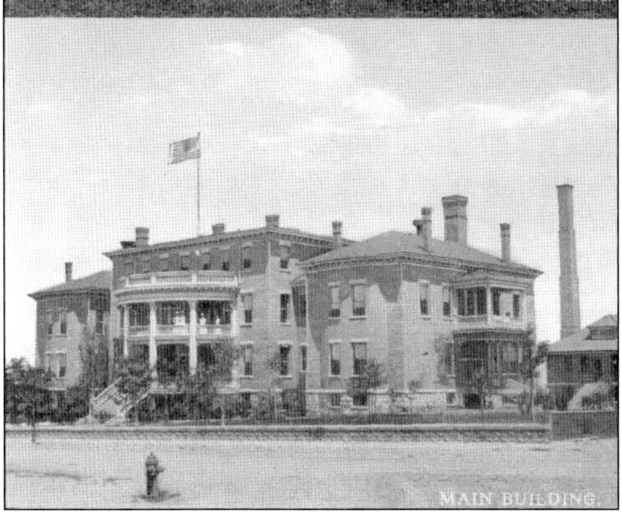

Most TB patients arrived in Albuquerque by train, although at least one arrived from Indiana in a chartered ambulance plane. Lungers at St. Joseph lived in either the san's main building or in one of 17 original cottages; a dozen more were added by 1919. Most patients, including, in the above photograph, Tom Johnson (left) and Horton Davis, enjoyed their days at St. Joseph, although some complained about a singing deliveryman and skating neighborhood kids who raised "a lot of racket during rest hours." In 1920, Grace Edmister complained that the screens on her cottage did not prevent sand from blowing in and covering her as she tried to rest. (Above, courtesy of the Albuquerque Museum, PA1993.17.25.)

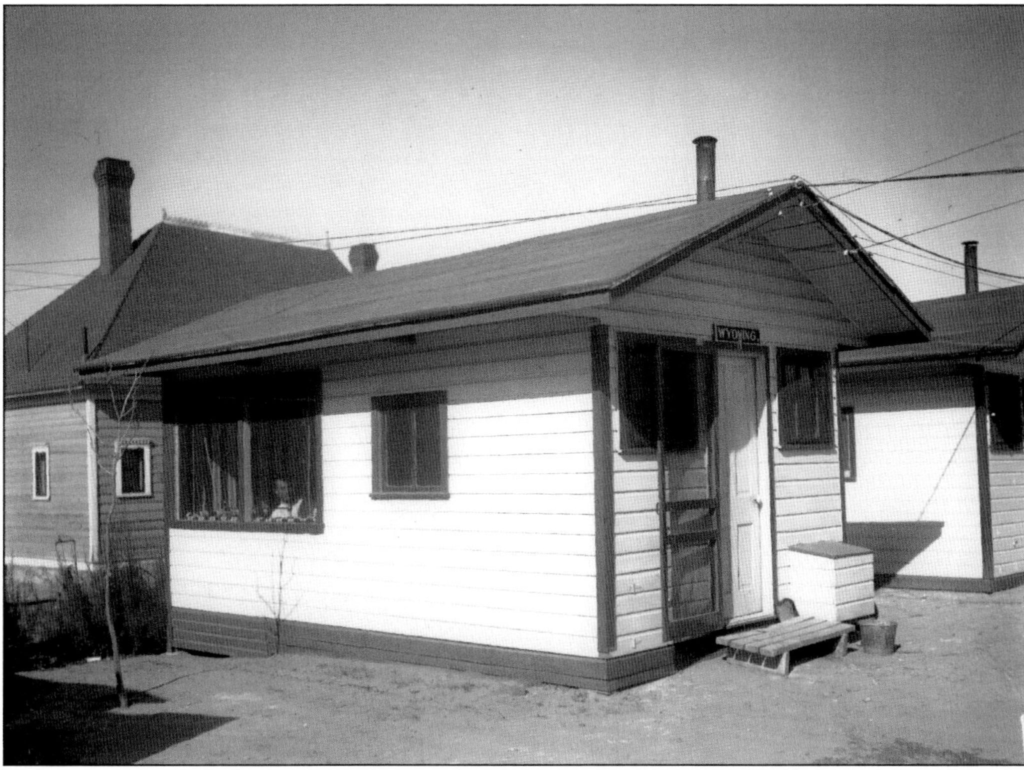

St. Joseph was the first san in Albuquerque designed in the "cottage plan," with tents (later wood-frame bungalows) built in rows north of the general hospital's main building. The arrangement reminded one observer of a mother hen surrounded by her chicks. According to the *Albuquerque Journal*, the cottages were "placed in such a position as to permit patients to enjoy sunshine nearly every day from early morning until late afternoon." (Above, courtesy of the Albuquerque Museum, PA1992.5.704.)

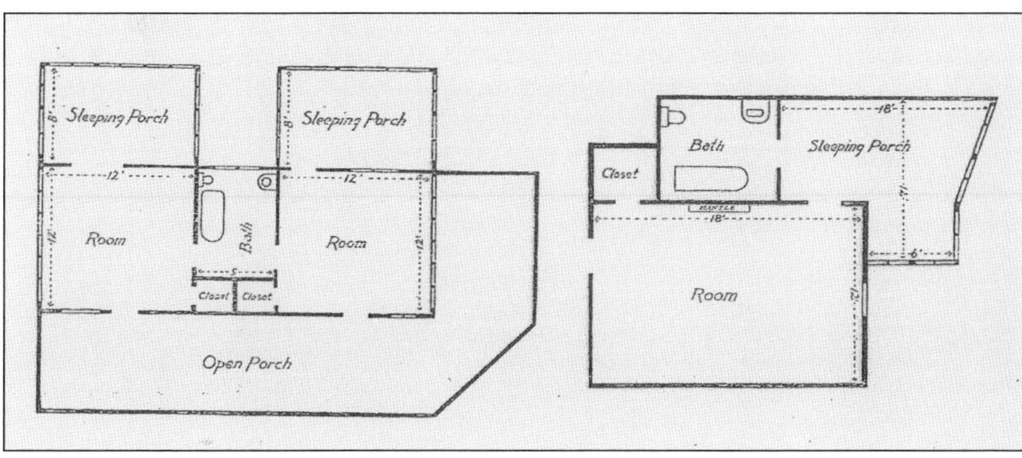

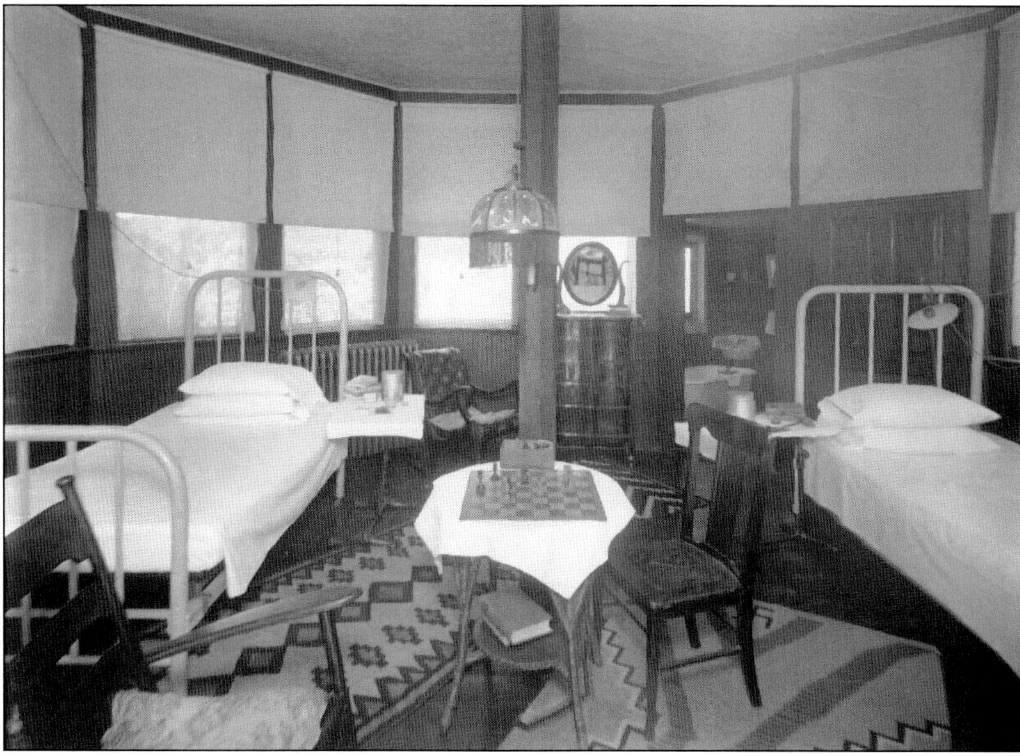

Most private cottages came with electricity, call bells, running water, steam heat, and large screened windows. As required by a territorial law of 1907, cottages were disinfected with the departure of each TB tenant. A cottage's main physical characteristic was its all-important sleeping porch, a feature that had become popular in middle-class homes by the early 20th century. (Above, courtesy of the Albuquerque Museum, PA1992.5.697; below, courtesy of Nancy Tucker.)

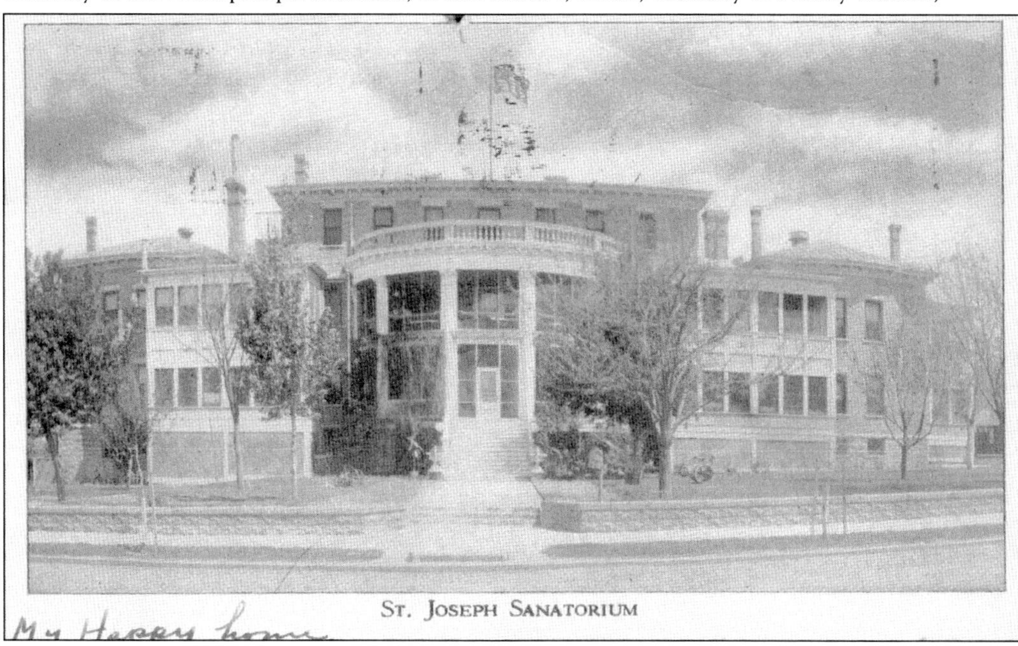

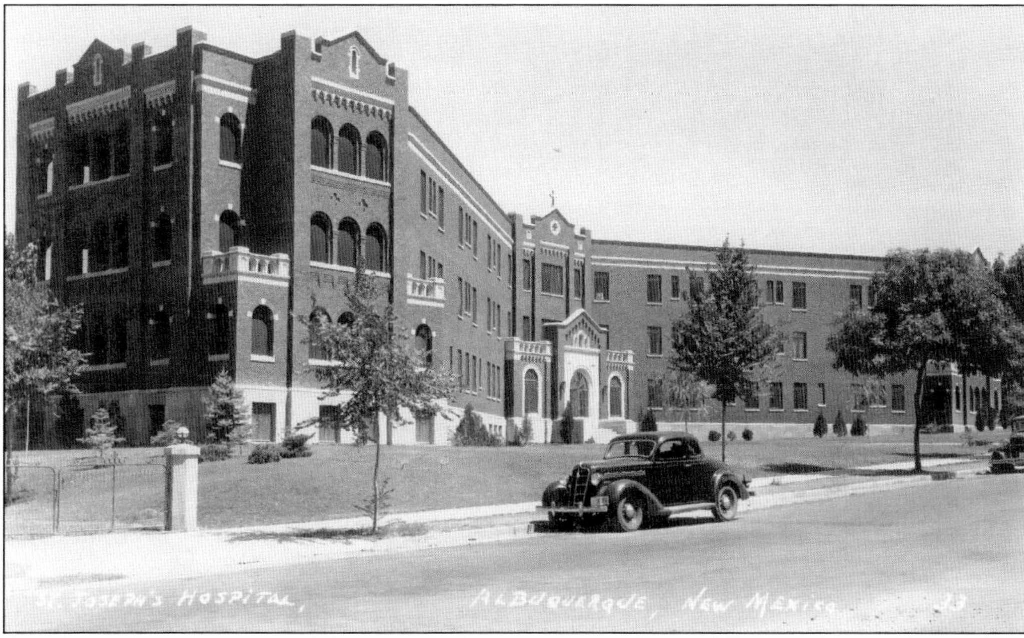

St. Joseph built a new, 150-bed general hospital, said to be the most modern in the Southwest, in 1930. The san's cottages were closed during the Great Depression, causing a migration of lungers to either the hospital's main building or to other sans, near and far. Many men and women cried as they watched wreckers destroy the last of the san's cottages in May 1939. The san's original building was demolished in 1968, with everything from a baby grand piano to tiled fireplaces auctioned off or given to Brother Matthias's Good Shepherd Refuge elsewhere in Albuquerque. (Both, courtesy of Jim Coad.)

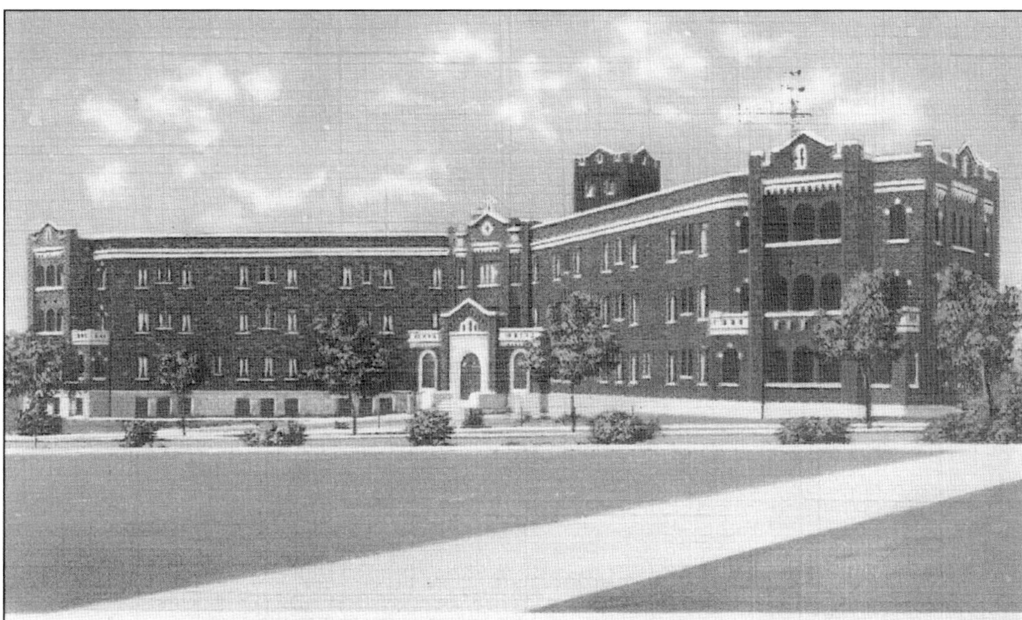

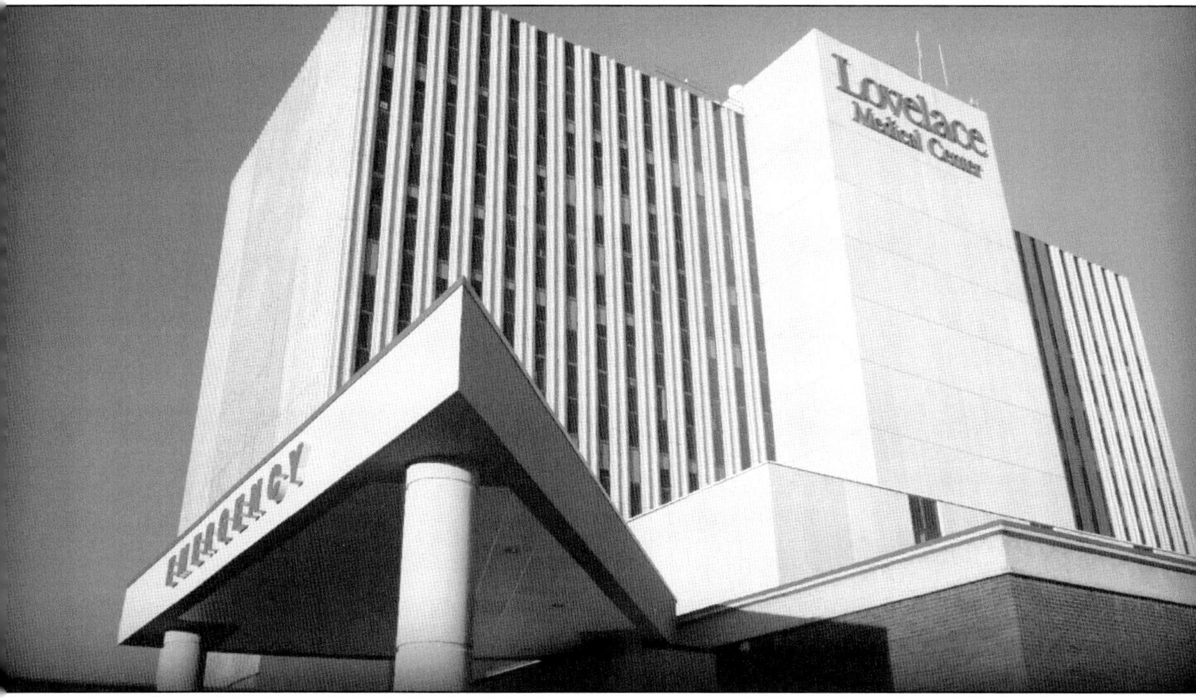

Still a major hospital, St. Joseph's "thoroughly modern" general hospital of 1930 was replaced by a state-of-the-art facility in 1967. Sold in 2003, the 1967 building is now the 10-story, 263-bed Lovelace Medical Center. The 1930 building is still part of the greater hospital complex. (Courtesy of the Lovelace Health System.)

Four

Albuquerque's Presbyterian Sanatorium

The idea of a Presbyterian Sanatorium in Albuquerque was the brainchild of Rev. Hugh Albert Cooper. After 15 years of service as a minister of Presbyterian churches in the Midwest, Cooper came to Albuquerque as a health-seeker in 1903. Regaining his health, Cooper became the pastor of Albuquerque's First Presbyterian Church in 1904.

Cooper noted that with only one sanatorium (St. Joseph) in his new community, care for residents with TB was "woefully inadequate." Many lungers lived on their own, in poverty and without adequate medical care. Entire families occupied one-room rented shacks or tents on the south ends of Arno, Edith, and Walter Streets. Other lungers lived in a "tent city" at Mountain Road and North Tenth Street. Agreeing with Cooper that something needed to be done to assist destitute lungers, a committee of nine members from the Presbyterian Church's Synod of New Mexico traveled to Santa Fe and other towns of the territory in search of the best location to build a new san. The committee concluded that Albuquerque offered the ideal climate, property, and potential space for future expansion.

The synod's first small san was located in a five-room residence on the corner of Central Avenue and Oak Street. The synod purchased the property for $4,000. A new, enlarged facility opened with a main building, five cottages, and two initial patients on August 1, 1908. Dr. S.G. Sewell joined the san's medical staff and moved four small cottages he had built to the new Presbyterian san at 1012 East Central Avenue. Presbyterian's first building boom had begun. With only short periods of respite, the expansion has never ceased.

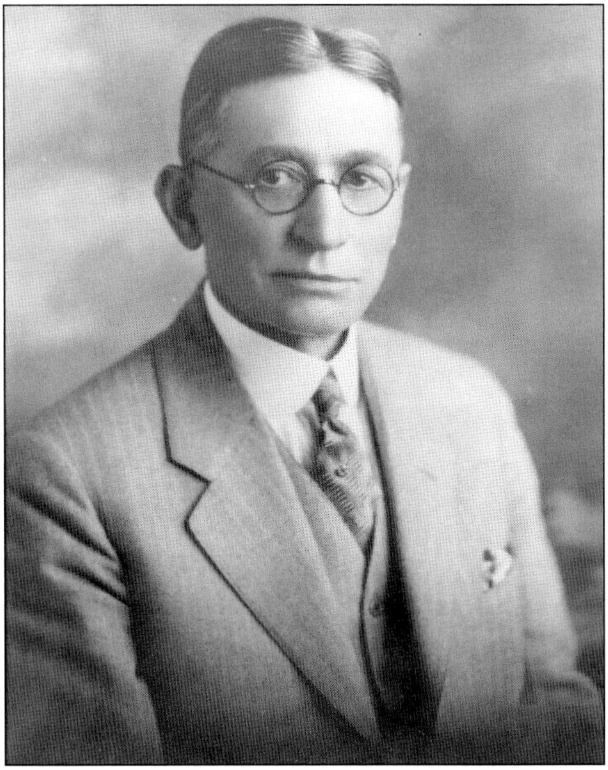

Rev. Hugh Cooper played many roles in Albuquerque's TB community. In addition to founding the Presbyterian Sanatorium and raising funds for its maintenance and growth, he also ministered to many of his patients' spiritual needs, in good times and in bad. He officiated at many weddings and, sadly, presided over many funerals when lungers succumbed, having failed in their quests for a cure. (Courtesy of Presbyterian Healthcare Services.)

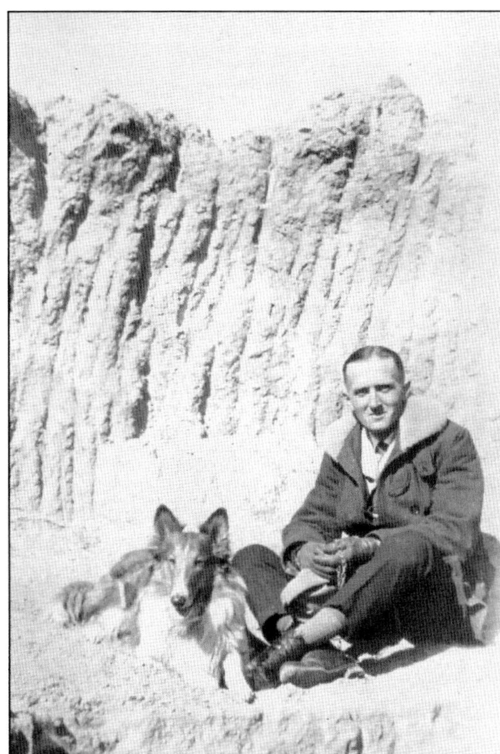

The Reverend Cooper was ably assisted by many employees, but especially by Marion Kellogg, who came to the san from New York to be with her fiancé, lunger Jimmie Van Devanter (pictured with their dog, Fuzzy). Despite Van Devanter's failing health, the couple married in 1922. Their happy marriage lasted seven years, until Jimmie's death in 1929. (Courtesy of Presbyterian Healthcare Services.)

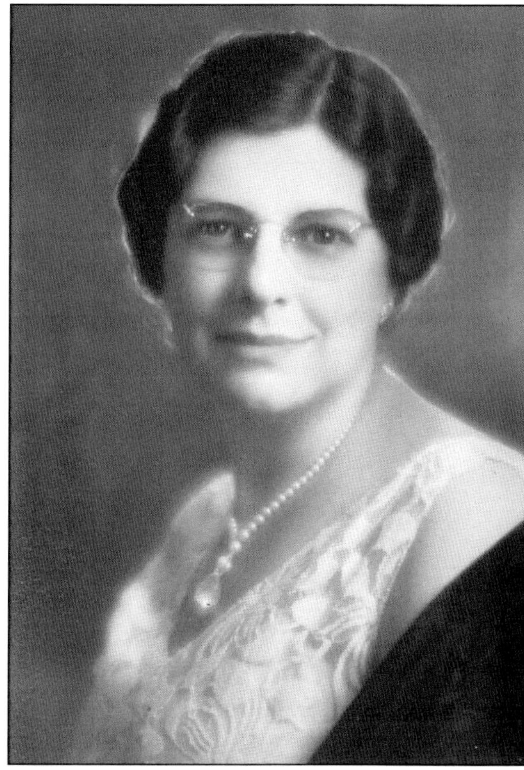

Rev. Cooper's wife, Delia, hired Marion Kellogg (right) as the san's secretary in 1921. She was soon involved in nearly every facet of the san's operation, especially when Rev. Cooper was away on long fundraising trips back East. Kellogg was the ideal person for such a varied job. Although born into an affluent family, she had always "yearned to serve," as historian Mo Palmer puts it. "Mrs. Van," as she was universally known after her marriage, did everything at Presbyterian, from visiting patients (leaving notes of encouragement on their trays) to editing the san's long-running newsletter. Her workload increased even more with Rev. Cooper's death from a heart attack in 1934. Mrs. Van worked at Presbyterian and served its patients, her "children," for over 50 years. She died at age 91 in 1984. (Right, courtesy of Presbyterian Healthcare Services.)

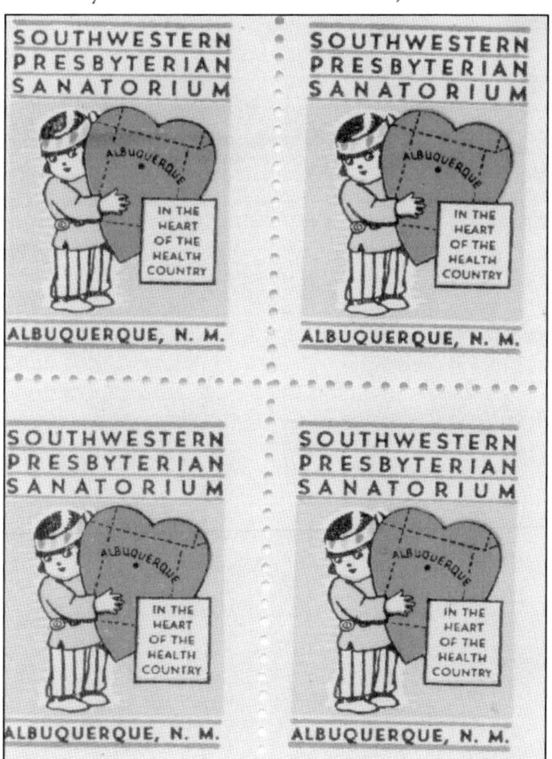

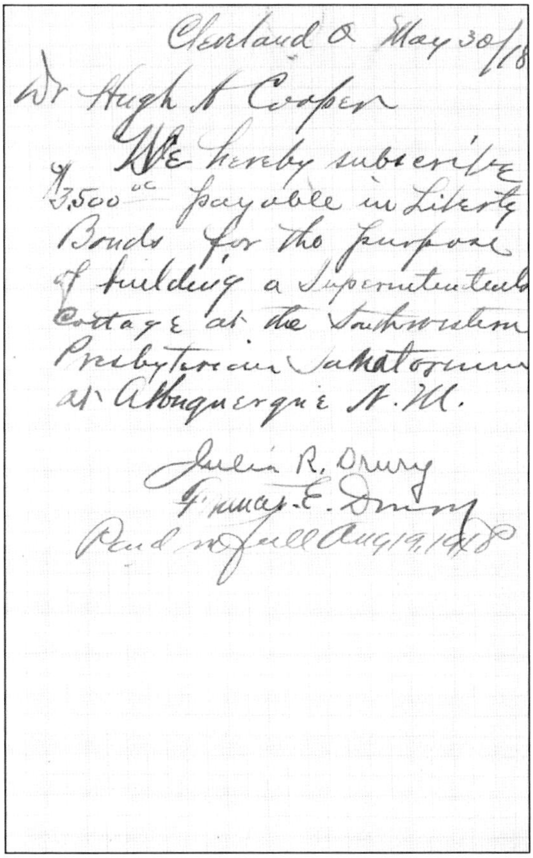

Cleveland O May 30/18
Dr Hugh A Cooper
We hereby subscribe
$3,500.00 payable in Liberty
Bonds for the purpose
of building a Superintendents
Cottage at the Southwestern
Presbyterian Sanatorium
at Albuquerque N.M.
Julia R. Drury
Francis E. Drury
Paid in full Aug 19, 1918

Fearing fires, Rev. Cooper worked to replace tents with more permanent cottages as soon as possible. To raise money for this construction, Cooper often named cottages and whole buildings after generous benefactors. Mrs. Cyrus H. McCormick, for example, donated $6,000 ($91,000 in today's money) for a new structure, named the McCormick Building. When Presbyterian ministers contributed money for a building where they and their families could receive care if they contracted TB, the new facility was appropriately named the Ministers Building. Julia and Francis Drury contributed $3,500 ($53,000 today) for the Drury cottage (pictured below). They had contributed to the construction of a similar "cure cottage" at Saranac Lake, New York. Thanks to donations like these, Presbyterian had 6 large buildings, 23 cottages, and 150 patients by 1931. (Both, courtesy of Presbyterian Healthcare Services.)

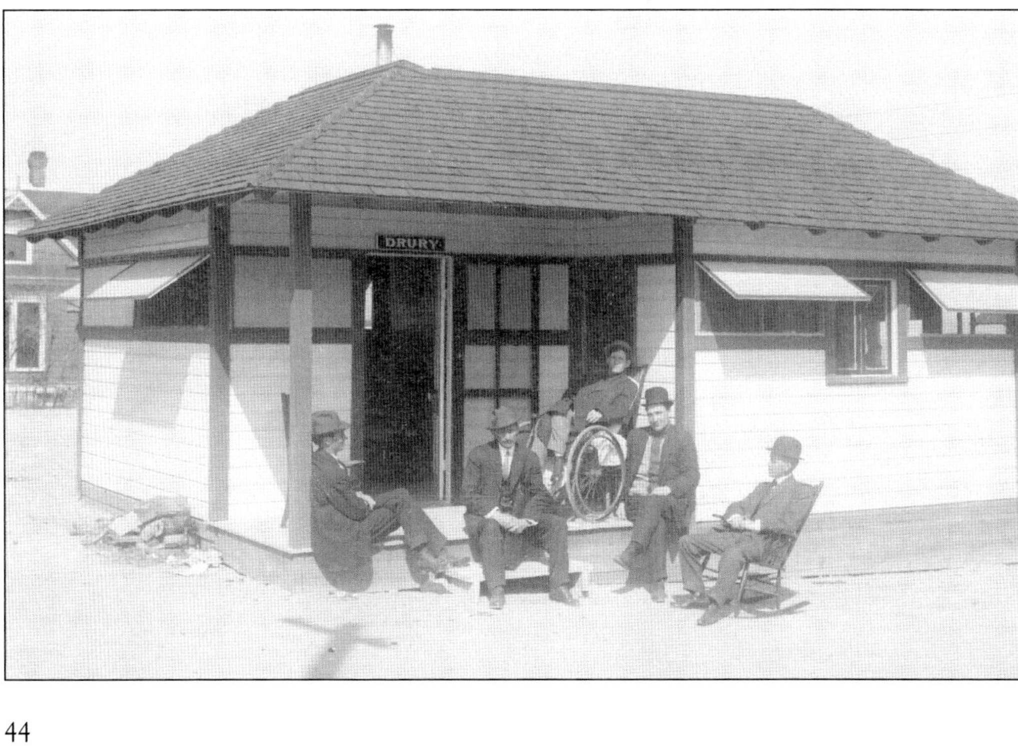

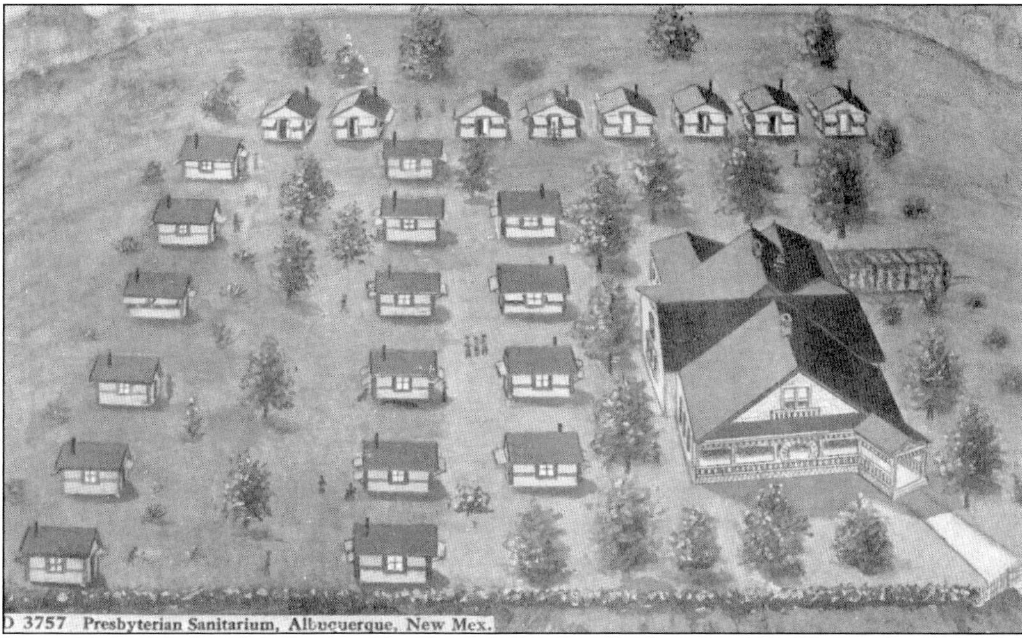

With vines, flowers, and well-kept lawns placed in a tranquil setting, cottages resembled small versions of Eastern middle-class houses, making transplants from that part of the country feel more at home, comfortable, and likely to be cured. (Above, courtesy of Jim Coad; below, courtesy of the Albuquerque Museum, PA1978.151.557.)

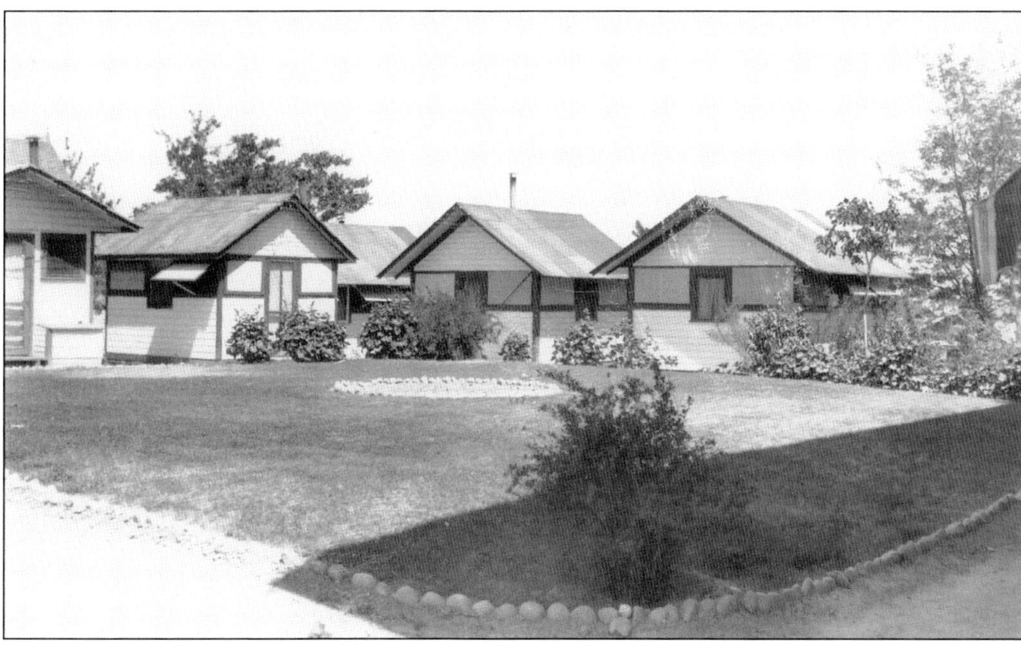

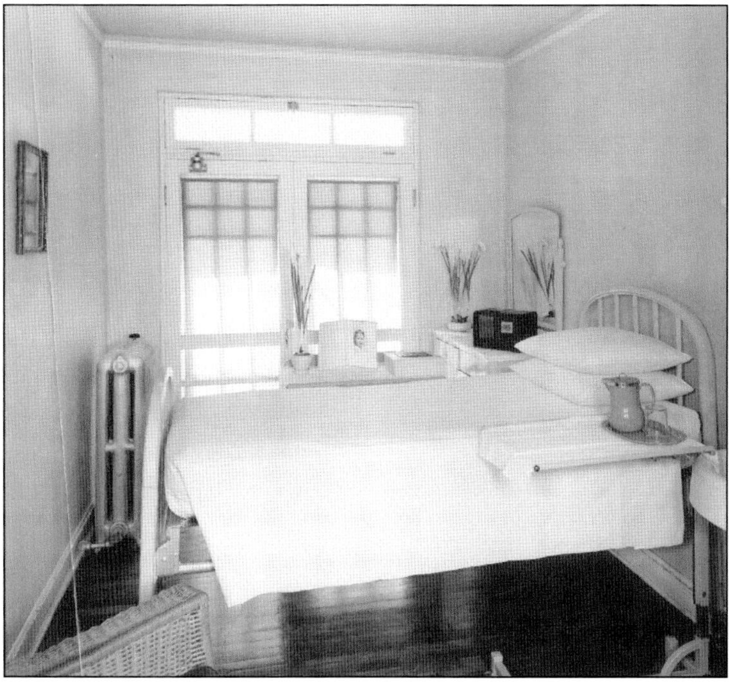

If reading was the patients' number one distraction, writing was number two. Patients corresponded with friends, relatives, and pen pals; one prolific patient mailed an average of five letters a day. Many lungers enthusiastically entered writing contests for small prizes. Verena Ream won $2.50 for her short story about a daydream in which she had "lots of fun" living without her doctor's restrictive rules. (Courtesy of Presbyterian Healthcare Services.)

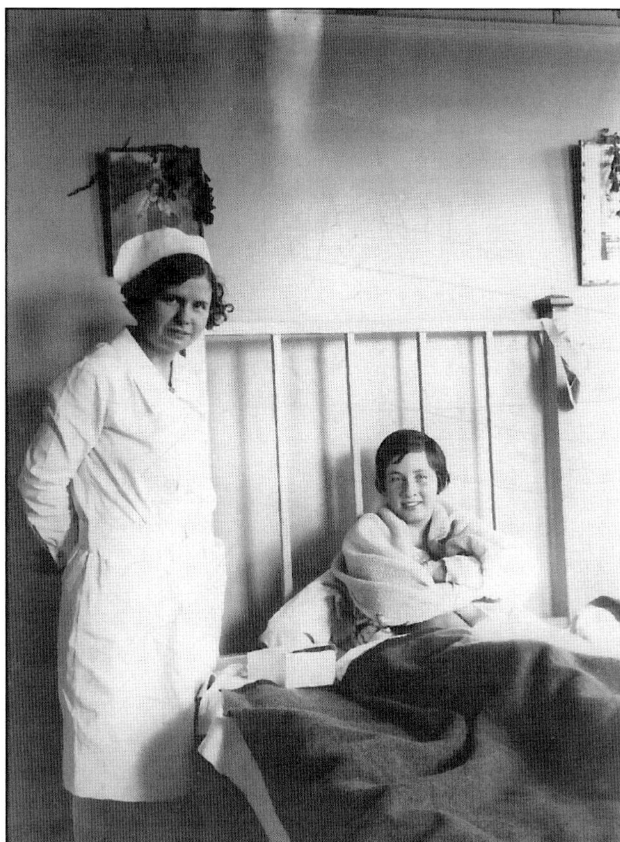

Presbyterian's youngest lunger, Mary Helen Alburt, was only nine when she caught TB. Although Presbyterian did not admit anyone younger than 18, Mrs. Van made an exception for Mary Helen when the girl and her mother arrived at the san in 1931. Mary Helen recovered, in part because of the extra attention she received from Mrs. Van, her nurses, tray boys, and fellow patients. (Courtesy of Presbyterian Healthcare Services.)

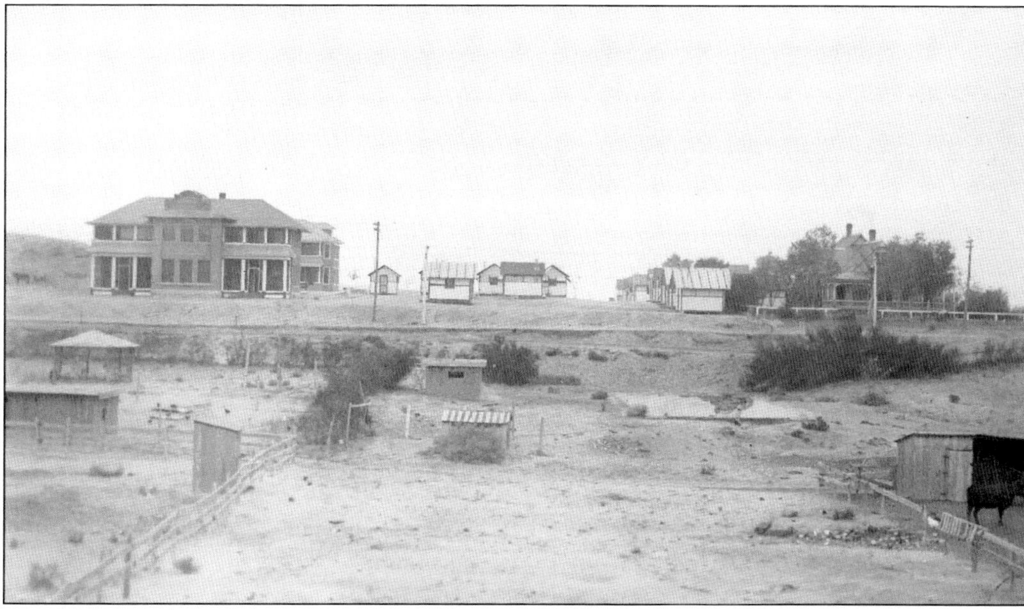

Like all hospital patients, lungers usually looked forward to visits from family members or friends. For a few moments, they could enjoy themselves and put their troubles on hold. Good visits were like balms, applied to temporarily soothe, although not necessarily heal, TB. Some patients, however, preferred to refuse or delay visits. In November 1913, Helen Norine, a teenage patient at St. Joseph's san in Silver City, wrote to her mother in Minnesota that she did not want "anyone to come down for Xmas cause I won't be well enough to be out of bed." Helen preferred that "someone come later on when I'm up and can go for a ride . . . for fun." Helen survived through Christmas alone, but died shortly after the new year. (Both, courtesy of Presbyterian Healthcare Services.)

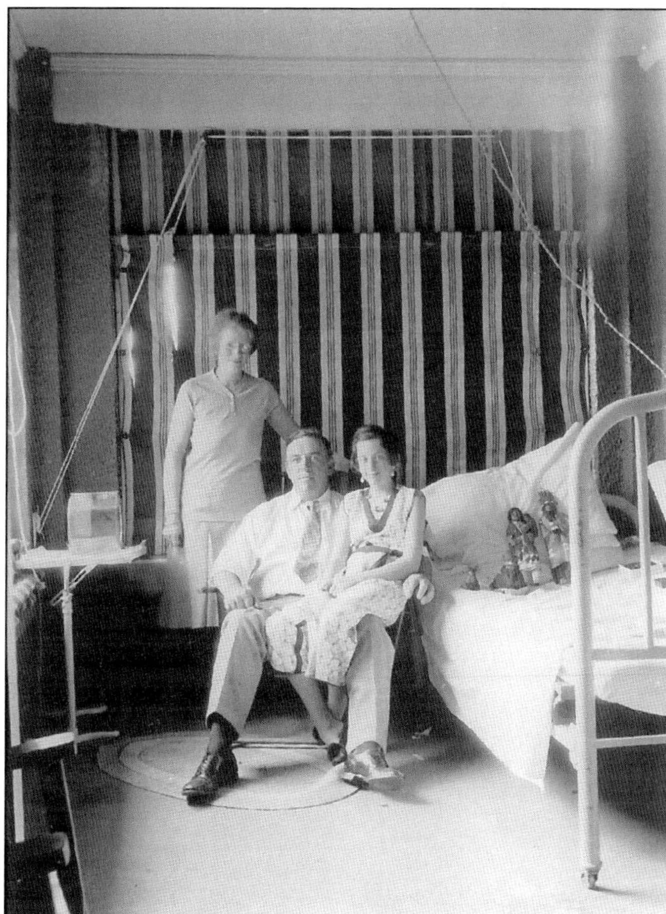

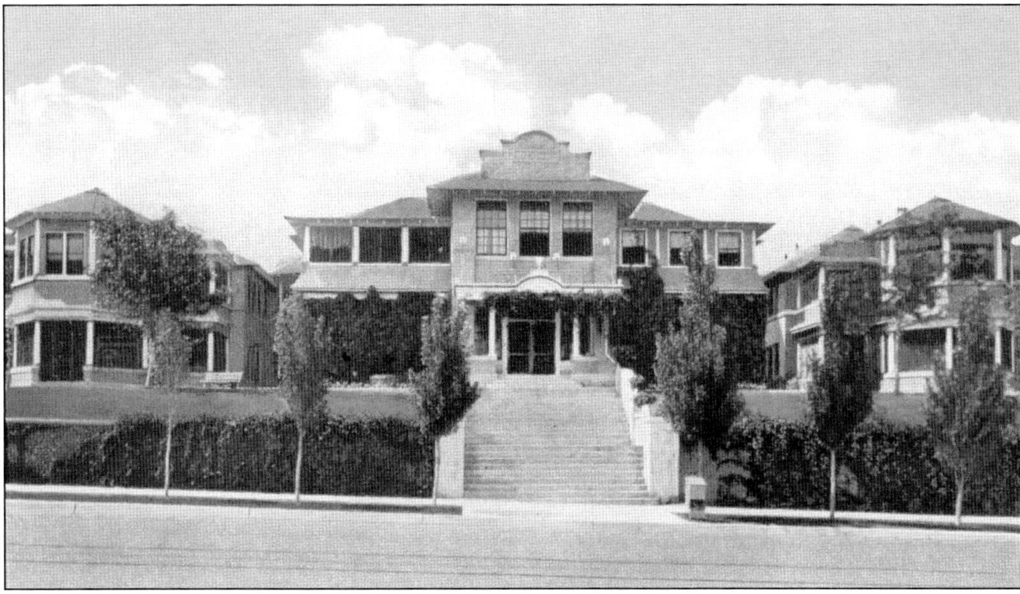

When Freda Lucille Maytag contracted TB and entered Presbyterian as a patient, her father, washing machine manufacturer Frederick L. Maytag, donated $150,000 for the building of a research facility to help find a cure for Freda's disease. The san agreed to raise $350,000 for research to be done in the new lab. Maytag Research Lab (below) was built by 1933, but Presbyterian failed to raise its share of research money at the height of the Great Depression. Upset by the lack of progress toward a cure for TB, Maytag sued the san; his legal action ended with his death in 1937. Freda lived to be 61. The Maytag building still stands, one of the only structures of the early san that remains at Presbyterian today. (Above, courtesy of Jim Coad; below, courtesy of Presbyterian Healthcare Services.)

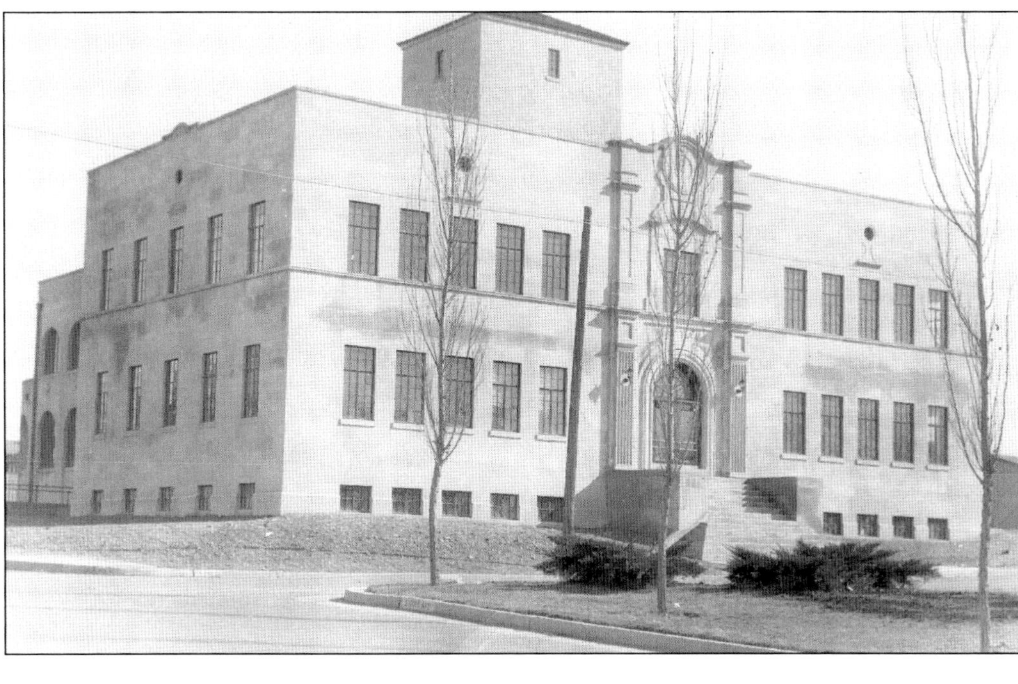

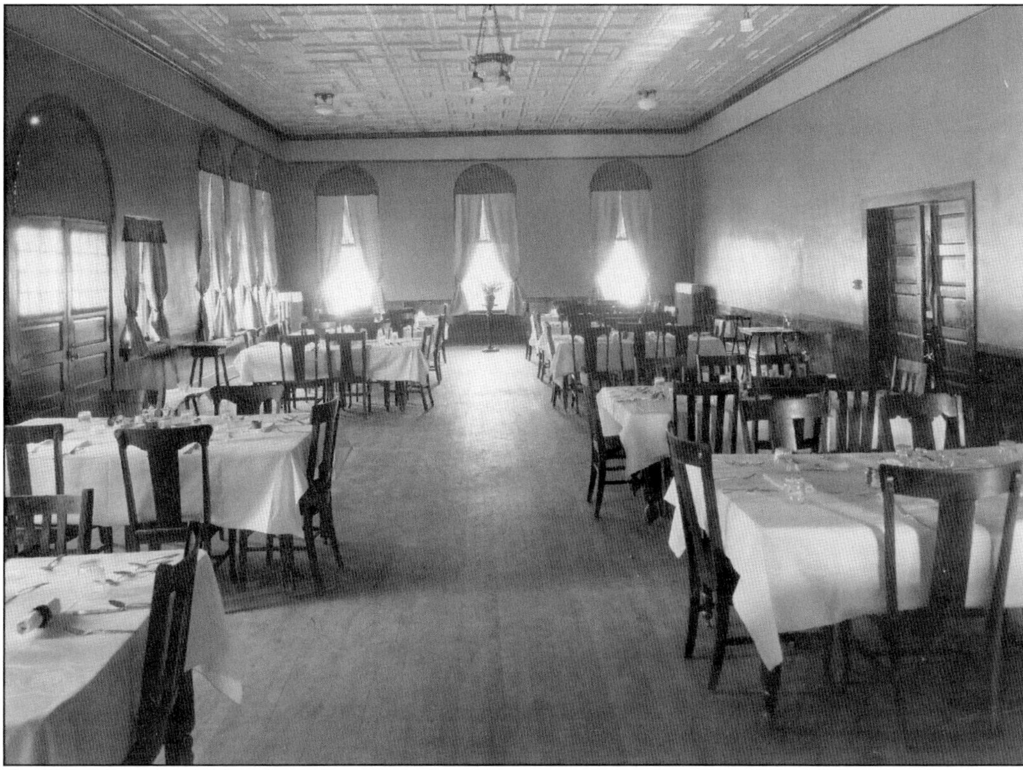

Presbyterian's proximity to Albuquerque's railroad station helped facilitate the transport of food and supplies to the san. Except at sans that grew much of their own food, food shortages and rationing during World War II were difficult on cooks preparing food for patients with their carefully monitored diets. Several sans grew victory gardens to help in the crisis. Presbyterian's 100-acre farm north of town had closed years earlier. War news was always a hot topic at dining rooms, including Presbyterian's (above). (Both, courtesy of Presbyterian Healthcare Services.)

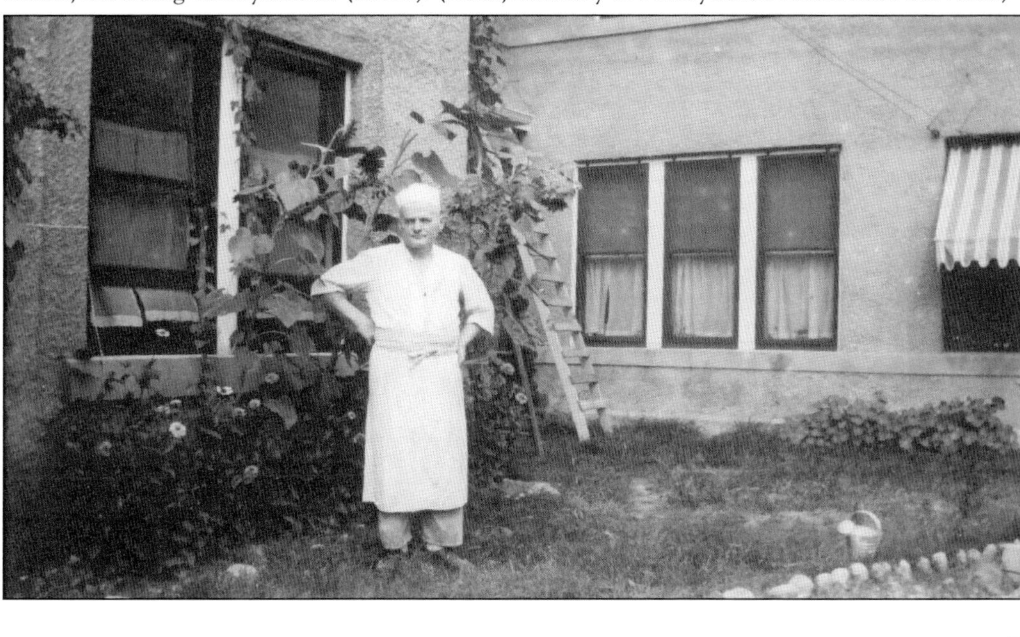

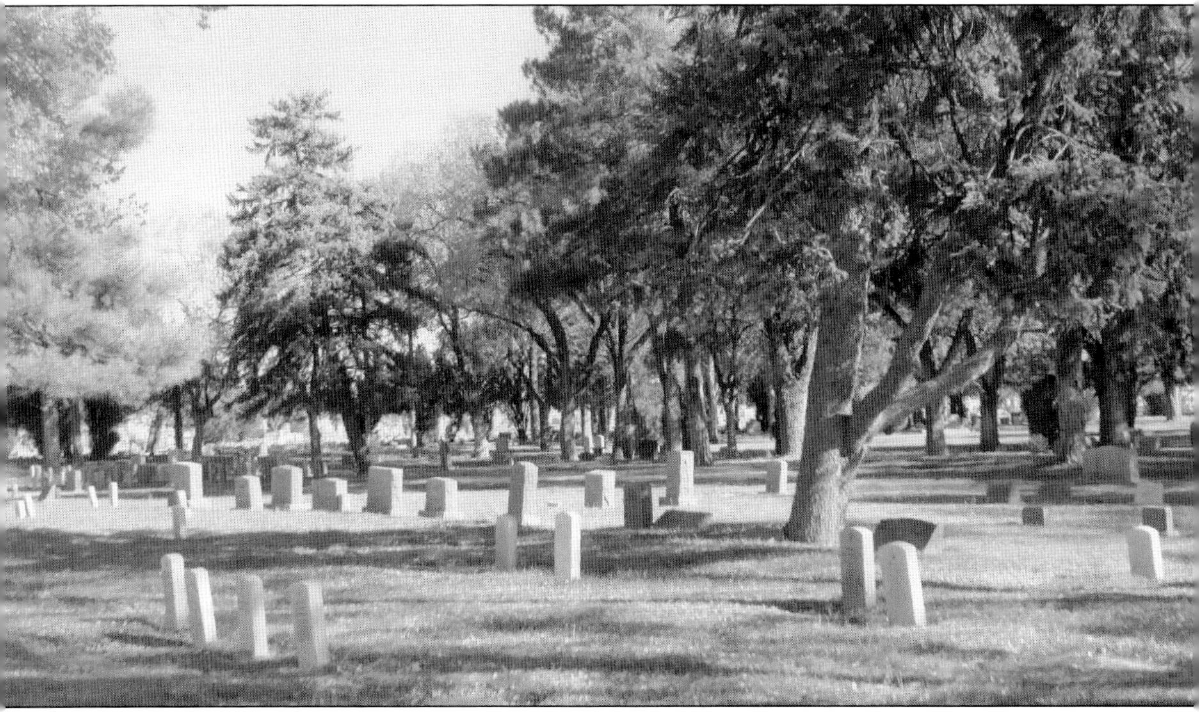

Death or the fear of death was the proverbial elephant in the room at all sans. John Duran recalls that he could recognize fellow lungers by their coughs, which became progressively worse as their TB advanced. Silence was a death knell. To lessen the impact on other patients, staff members closed a dead patient's door and waited until rest hours before removing the remains. Bodies were often buried in local cemeteries like Sunset, Mount Calvary, and Fairview (pictured here). A survey of 2,950 Fairview Cemetery burial records shows that TB remained the main cause of death (25 percent of the total) between 1881 and 1920. The average age of those who died of TB was only 34. The bodies of TB patients who had come to New Mexico from other states were transported home on trains. Family members often encountered complications en route, causing more stress and heartache for relatives, as happened to Mrs. Van, when she brought her husband's body home to be buried in Virginia in 1929.

Five

Albuquerque's Smaller Sanatoriums

While nearly every large town in New Mexico insisted that it had the best climate in the world to cure TB, town boosters in Albuquerque, with its fine climate and major railroad connections, made the greatest efforts to claim that their city was truly the "heart of the well country."

Albuquerque's Commercial Club (forerunner of the city's chamber of commerce) created a well-financed Civic Council to promote its healthcare industry. The council devised appealing slogans, including "Why Sacrifice Health for Wealth When Albuquerque Has Both?" The council launched national advertising campaigns, with slick promotions that appeared in popular middle-class magazines, like *Better Homes and Gardens*. Addressing doctors who might send their patients to Albuquerque, the council spent $14,000 (in today's money) for a year's worth of advertising in the *Journal of the American Medical Association* in 1917 alone.

The business community's efforts paid immediate dividends. Albuquerque soon became the health-seekers' primary destination in New Mexico and one of the main health-seeker destinations in the country. One TB expert estimated that by 1915, about one out of every five of Albuquerque's 11,020 residents were lungers.

While many newcomers lived on their own, more affluent health-seekers sought care in sanatoriums. Starting with St. Joseph and Presbyterian, the city's sans grew to include a second tier of smaller sans, such as the 50-bed Monbridge Manor, as well as a third tier of the smallest facilities, with 25 beds or less. In 1916, the Albuquerque Sanatorium charged as much as $135 per month, while sans with fewer amenities cost as little as $45 per month. Albuquerque's sans were created by private, religious, national, racial, and ethnic organizations. Health-care facilities like the VA hospital and the Atchison, Topeka & Santa Fe Railway Hospital included special wards for lungers.

Albuquerque's sans faced crises, especially fires and financial problems. Many sans closed after one or more emergencies, often reopening under new names and new ownership. Dr. Joseph S. Cipes's sanatorium thus became the Methodist Deaconess Sanatorium. Dr. A.G. Shortle's Albuquerque Sanatorium became the National Lutheran Sanatorium and then the AHEPA (American Hellenic Educational Progressive Association) Sanatorium. And Dr. W.T. Murphey's Sanatorium became St. John's Sanatorium and then the Hillcrest Sanatorium.

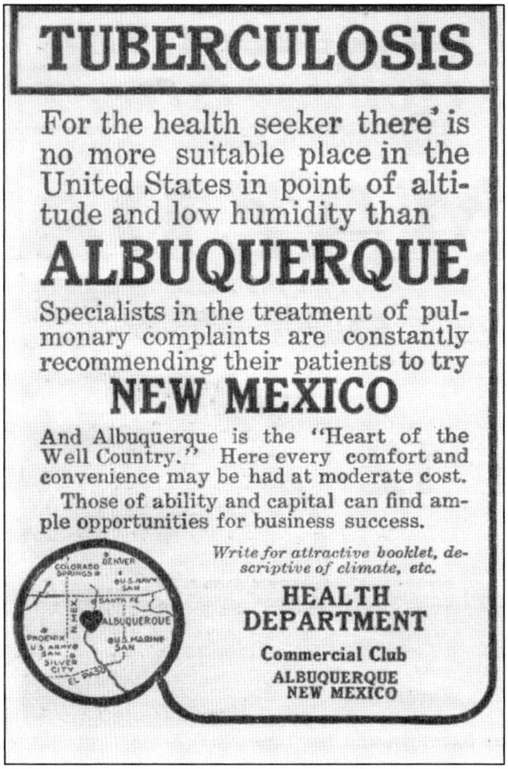

Advertisements like these appeared across the country. Recognizing the enormous potential profits of the health industry, other Southwestern states were not above advertising in New Mexico to lure away health-seekers. In 1916, the Prescott, Arizona, Chamber of Commerce advertised a special offer in the *Albuquerque Journal*, enticing lungers who craved "better climate, better water, better board, better cottages, better beds, [and] better treatment," all "free from sandstorms." The businessmen of Prescott were so confident, they promised free train fare back to New Mexico if a lunger was not satisfied with life in Arizona within 60 days. Many Albuquerque patients were known to at least winter in Tucson. To stem this tide, Albuquerque's *Health City Sun* printed a "weather report" that claimed that Tucson's weather was "lousy" and Phoenix's was "a darn site worse."

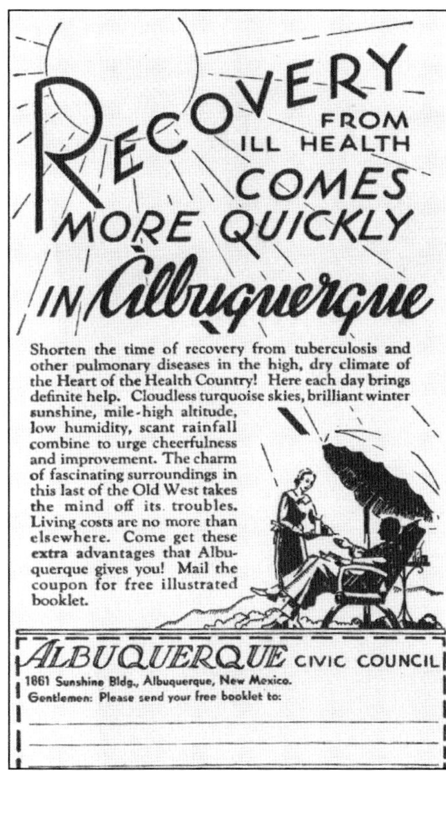
RECOVERY FROM ILL HEALTH COMES MORE QUICKLY IN Albuquerque
Shorten the time of recovery from tuberculosis and other pulmonary diseases in the high, dry climate of the Heart of the Health Country! Here each day brings definite help. Cloudless turquoise skies, brilliant winter sunshine, mile-high altitude, low humidity, scant rainfall combine to urge cheerfulness and improvement. The charm of fascinating surroundings in this last of the Old West takes the mind off its troubles. Living costs are no more than elsewhere. Come get these extra advantages that Albuquerque gives you! Mail the coupon for free illustrated booklet.
ALBUQUERQUE CIVIC COUNCIL
1861 Sunshine Bldg., Albuquerque, New Mexico.
Gentlemen: Please send your free booklet to:

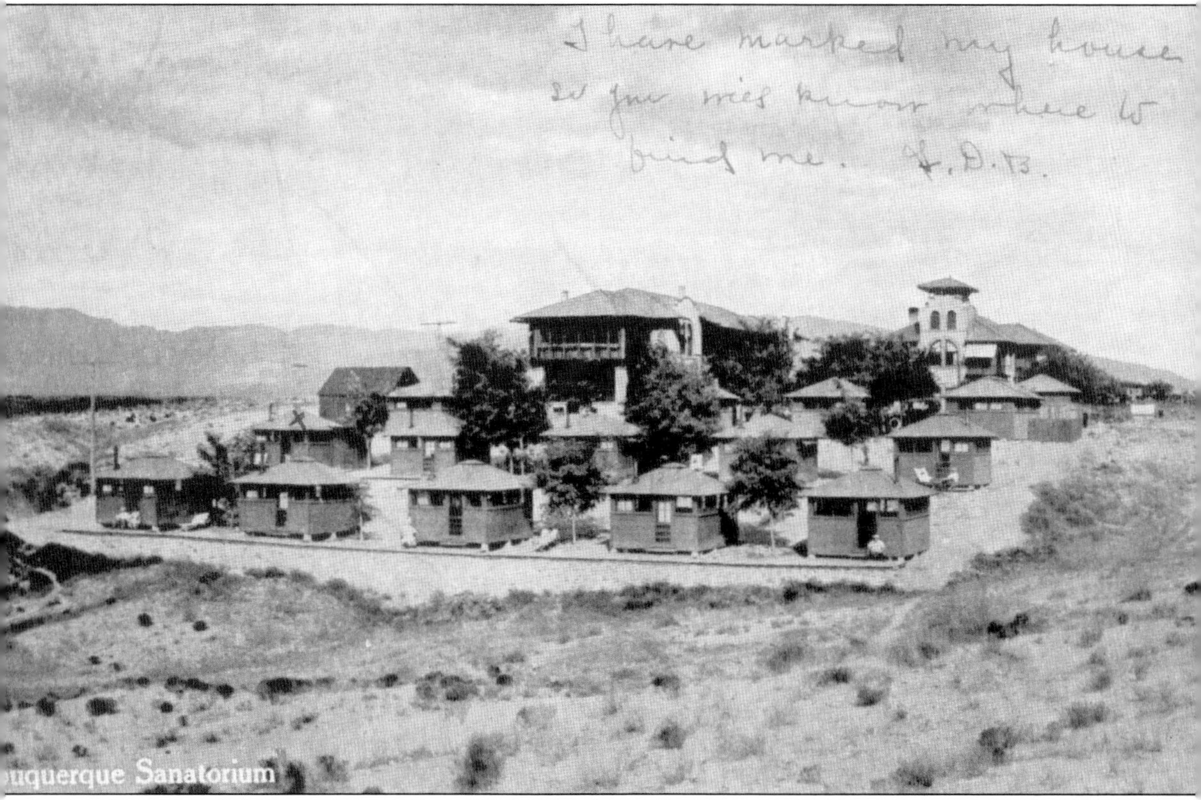

Dr. A.G. Shortle of Indiana completed his medical degree in 1896 and studied with the renowned chest specialist Dr. Carl Spengler in Davos, Switzerland. Dr. Shortle moved to Albuquerque in 1908, a victim of TB, the very disease he had studied. He soon recognized the need for a new san in Albuquerque, where only St. Joseph and Presbyterian offered care for lungers. Although he faced initial opposition from some who thought that such a san would harm the town and its reputation, Shortle persisted and opened his new Albuquerque Sanatorium in 1909. Touring the country to raise money and promote his san, Shortle was said to have helped prime the pump that brought an ever-increasing stream of health-seekers to Albuquerque. (Courtesy of Jim Coad.)

ALBUQUERQUE SANATORIUM

ALBUQUERQUE SANATORIUM

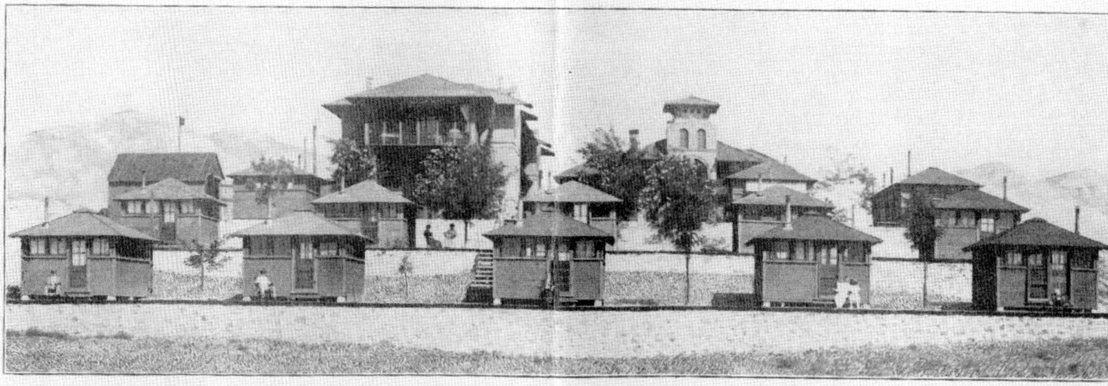

A. G. SHORTLE, M. D.
LE ROY S. PETERS, M. D.
Associate Physicians

M. W. AKERS
Superintendent

MRS. H. G. WEHKING
Matron

Sanatoriums produced handsome promotional brochures to attract health-seekers from across the country. The Albuquerque Sanatorium's brochure claims that, while the "famous resorts of the Alps" have the "beneficial results of altitude" and, while those in Phoenix and Tucson have a dry climate, Albuquerque has both. The brochure even boasts that "we have never seen a case of tuberculosis contracted by a [local] white person" in the city. (Courtesy of Nancy Tucker.)

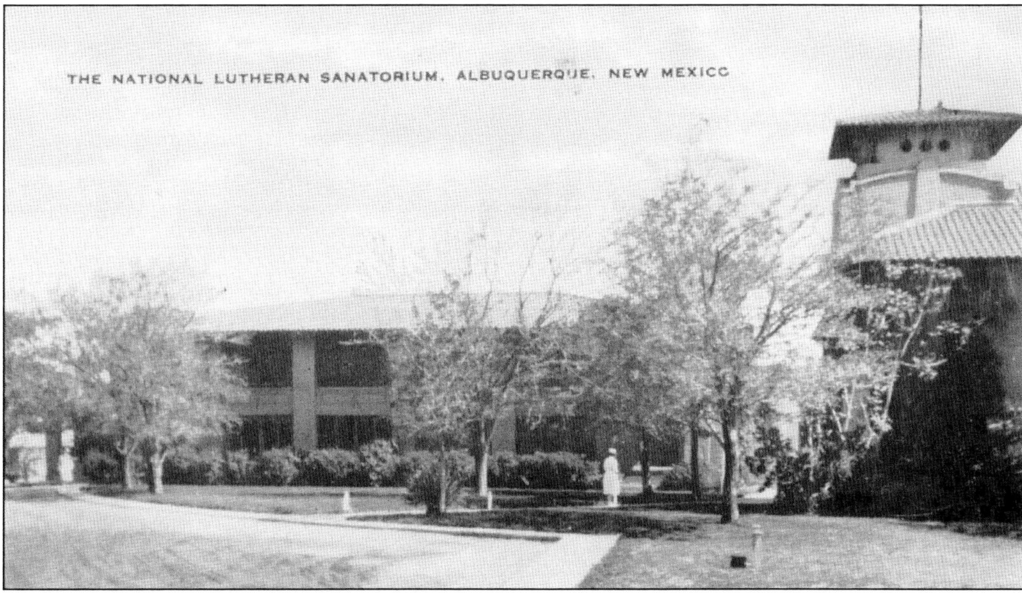

Dr. Shortle remained active with his san, his fundraising tours, and his writing until his death in 1922 at age 51. His san remained open until 1929, when it was sold to the Lutheran Church and became the National Lutheran Sanatorium. An open house was held for the san's reopening in April 1931, with many of the san's female patients wearing their best Sunday go-to-meeting pajamas. (Courtesy of Jim Coad.)

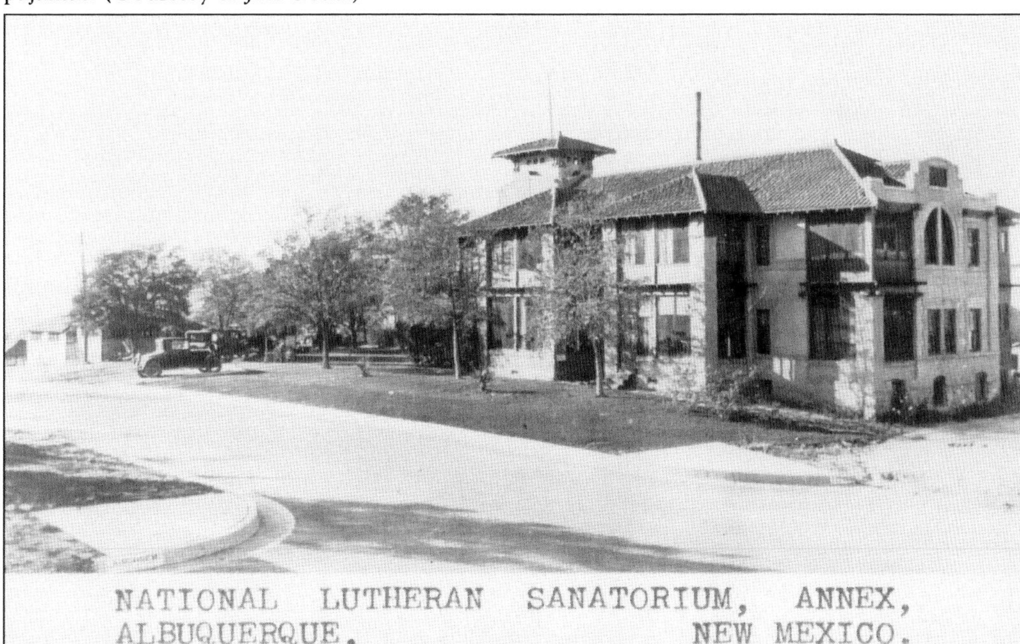

Advertisements for the new National Lutheran Sanatorium announced that suites in the san's main building cost $125 a month, while individual cottages cost $75 a month. These costs proved too expensive for many patients just as the nation faced the worst years of the Great Depression. In 1933, most of the san's remaining patients moved to nearby Presbyterian or St. Joseph, victims of "Old Man Depression" as well as of TB. (Courtesy of Nancy Tucker.)

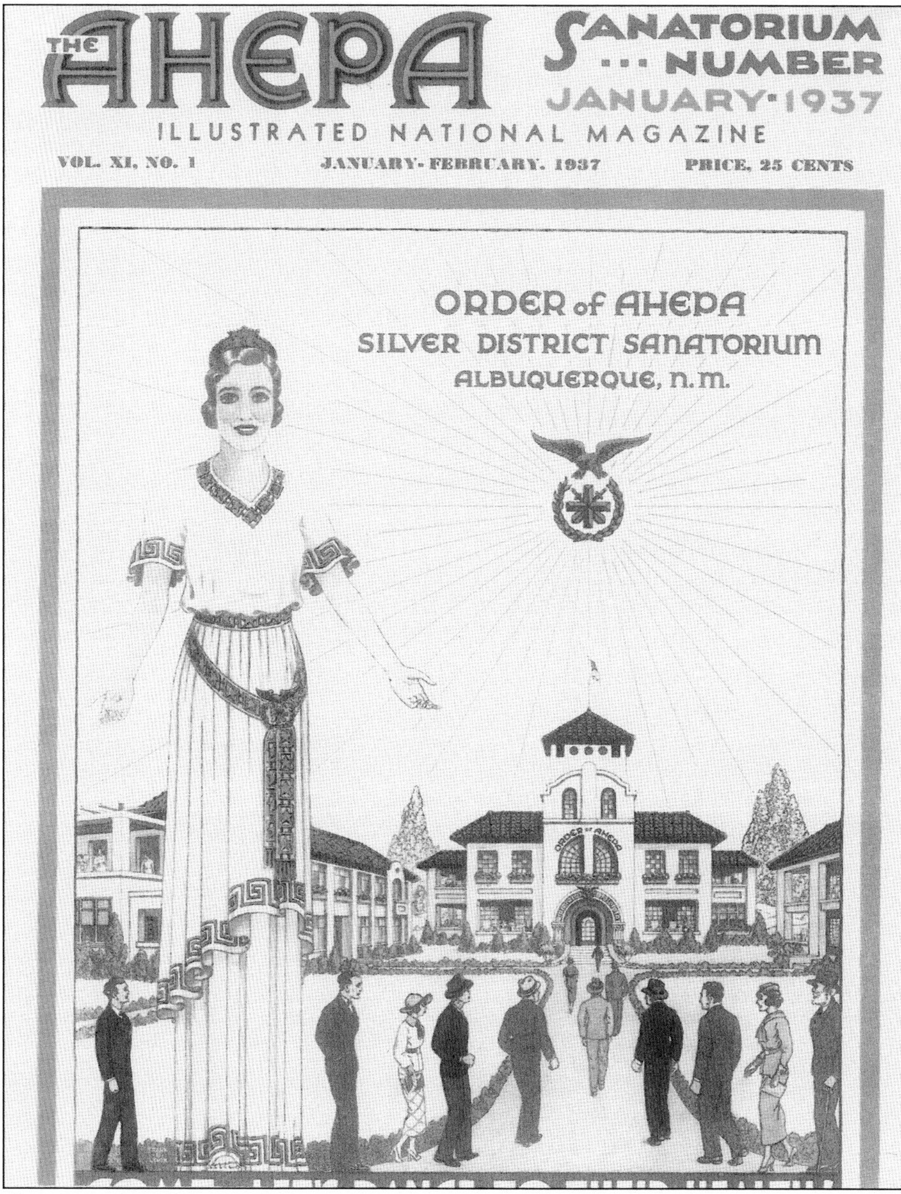

With four large buildings and six cottages, the former Albuquerque Sanatorium and National Lutheran Sanatorium was remodeled and reopened as the Order of AHEPA Silver District Tuberculosis Sanatorium on March 22, 1937, the anniversary of Greek independence. A high pontifical Greek Orthodox mass, a street parade, and other special events were organized to celebrate the day. To help create a "purely Hellenic environment," the san's first seven patients were treated to Greek cuisine by cook Peter Zoloumi. At its peak in 1940, the AHEPA San had 52 patients from 21 states. The san benefited from money raised at dances and other events held in Greek communities across the United States. In its promotional materials, the san vowed to provide a "relationship of host and guest rather than that of institution and patient." But the san reserved the right to refuse certain patients, having "no time, patience, or room for 'reds' or 'pinks' of any shade." (Courtesy of Katherine M. Pomonis.)

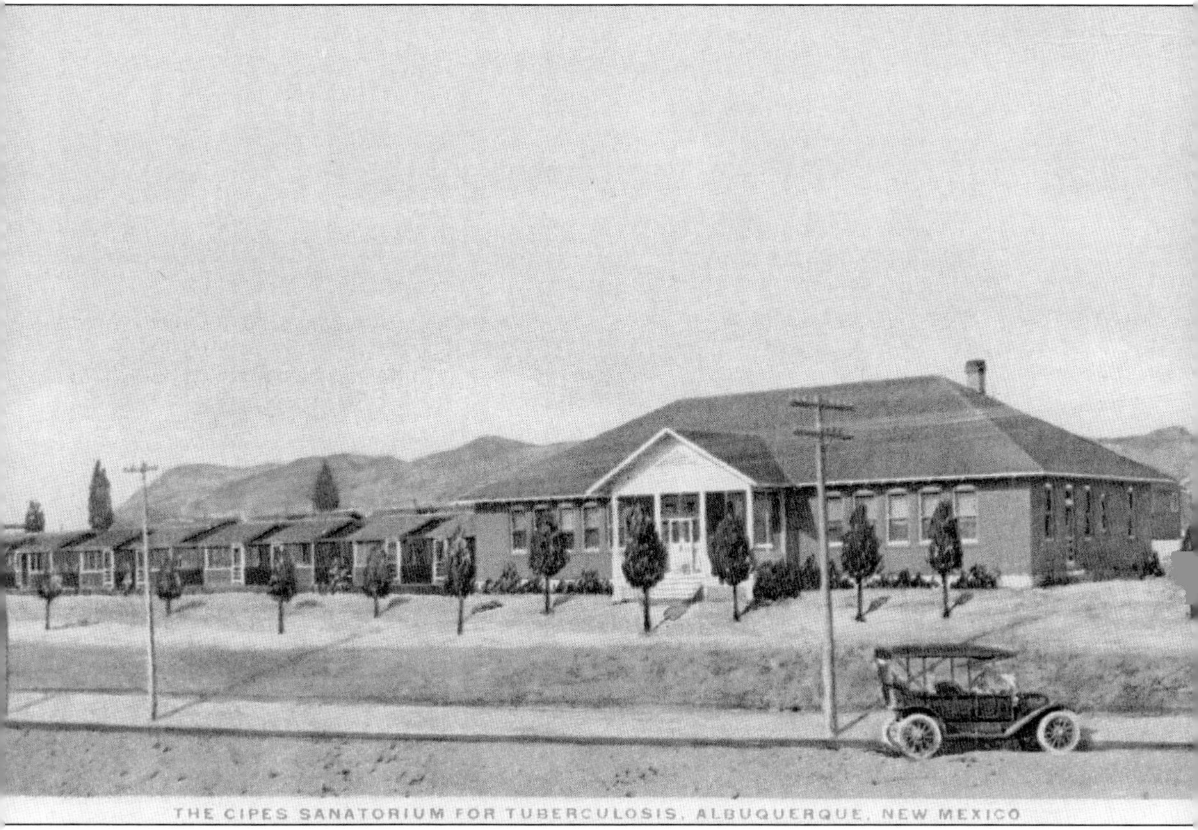

With the unanimous support of the Albuquerque Commercial Club, Dr. Joseph S. Cipes built a new san at 1631 East Central Avenue, just west of the University of New Mexico campus, in 1912. Costing more than $20,000 to construct, the san included a main building with an "especially attractive dining room" and eight "handsomely furnished" cottages, each with a closet and a bath, according to newspaper reports. Cipes's new san faced a minor fire in early 1913. Started in a linen closet about 6:00 a.m., the fire caused much smoke but little damage. Dr. Cipes later sold his property to the Methodist Woman's Home Missionary Society, which renamed it the Methodist Deaconess Sanatorium. (Courtesy of Jim Coad.)

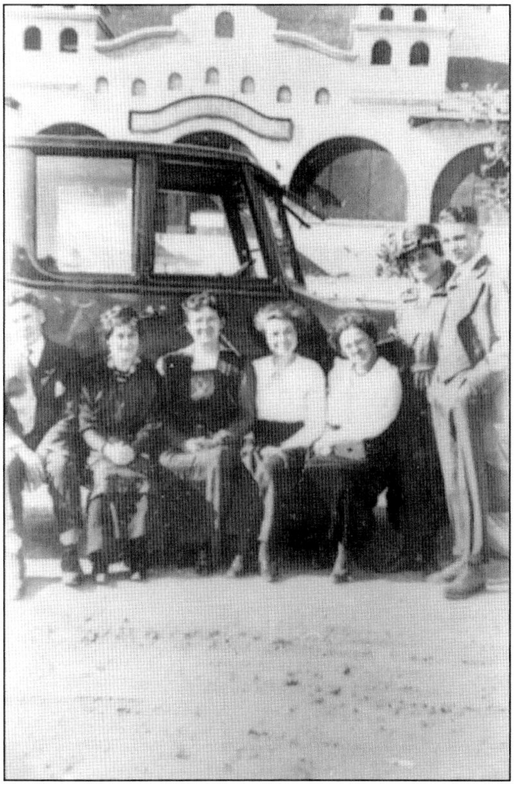

The Methodist Church's Woman's Home Missionary Society took over what had been Cipes's Sanatorium, renaming it the Methodist Deaconess Sanatorium. With help from New Mexico's famous Methodist missionary Thomas Harwood, the Woman's Home Missionary Society opened its successful san on Central Avenue. With time, so many sans lined Central Avenue that it became known as "lungers' alley." (Courtesy of the Albuquerque Museum, PA1993.26.3.)

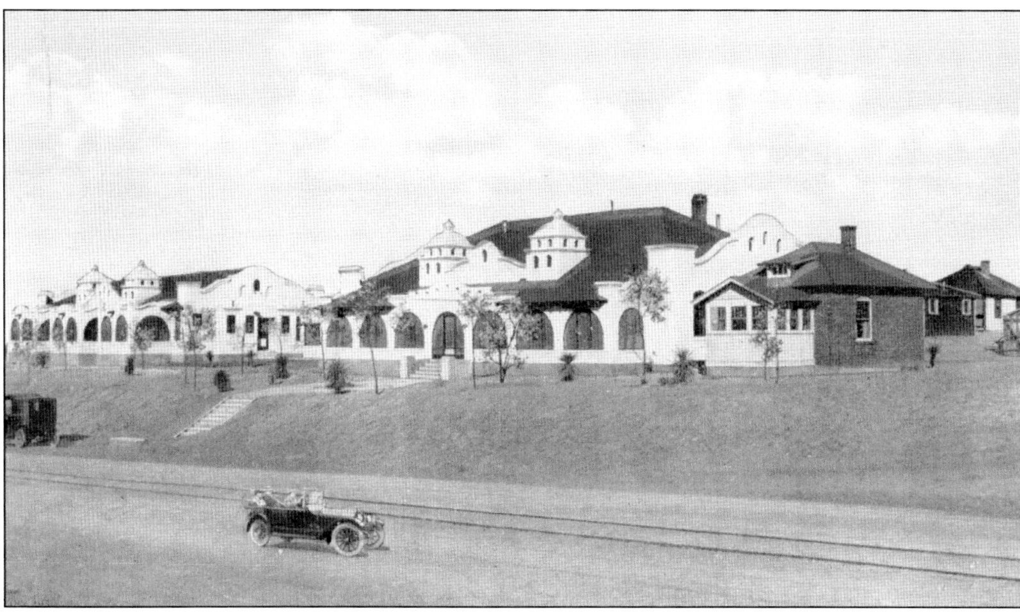

By 1919, Methodist Deaconess Sanatorium, redesigned in California Mission Revival style by Elson H. Norris, had admitted a total of 191 patients; 19 had been treated either free of charge or at reduced rates. By 1931, the san could accommodate 65 patients; by 1935, it had 50 cottages. Lungers came from across the United States and from such distant countries as China, Japan, and Ireland.

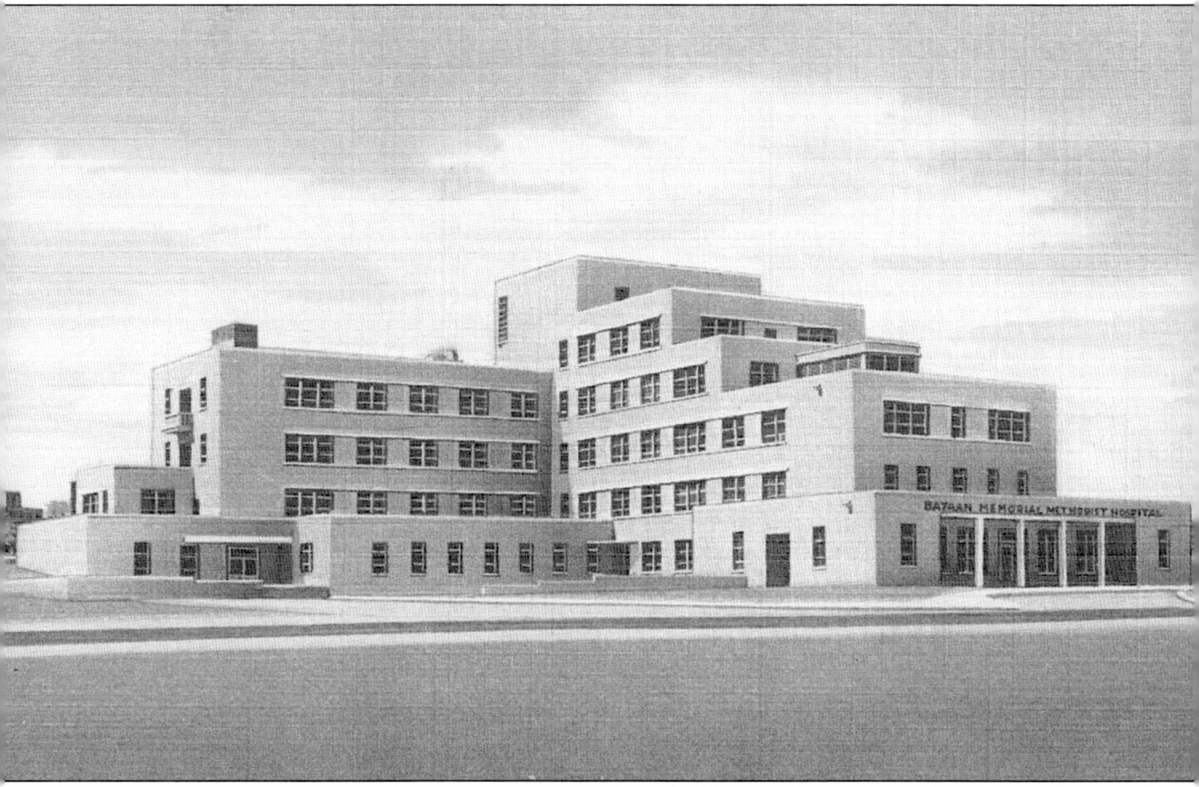

The Methodist Deaconess Sanatorium outlasted most other sans in Albuquerque, caring for lungers until 1949, when the Methodist Deaconess Society decided to take the institution in a new direction as a general hospital. Using land on Gibson Avenue donated by Dr. William Lovelace, the Bataan Memorial Methodist Hospital was designed in the Pueblo Revival style by former lunger John Gaw Meem. Construction began in 1950, with a grand opening in 1952. The hospital merged with the adjacent Lovelace Clinic in 1973, becoming, along with St. Joseph and Presbyterian, one of Albuquerque's three largest medical centers—all originally sans.

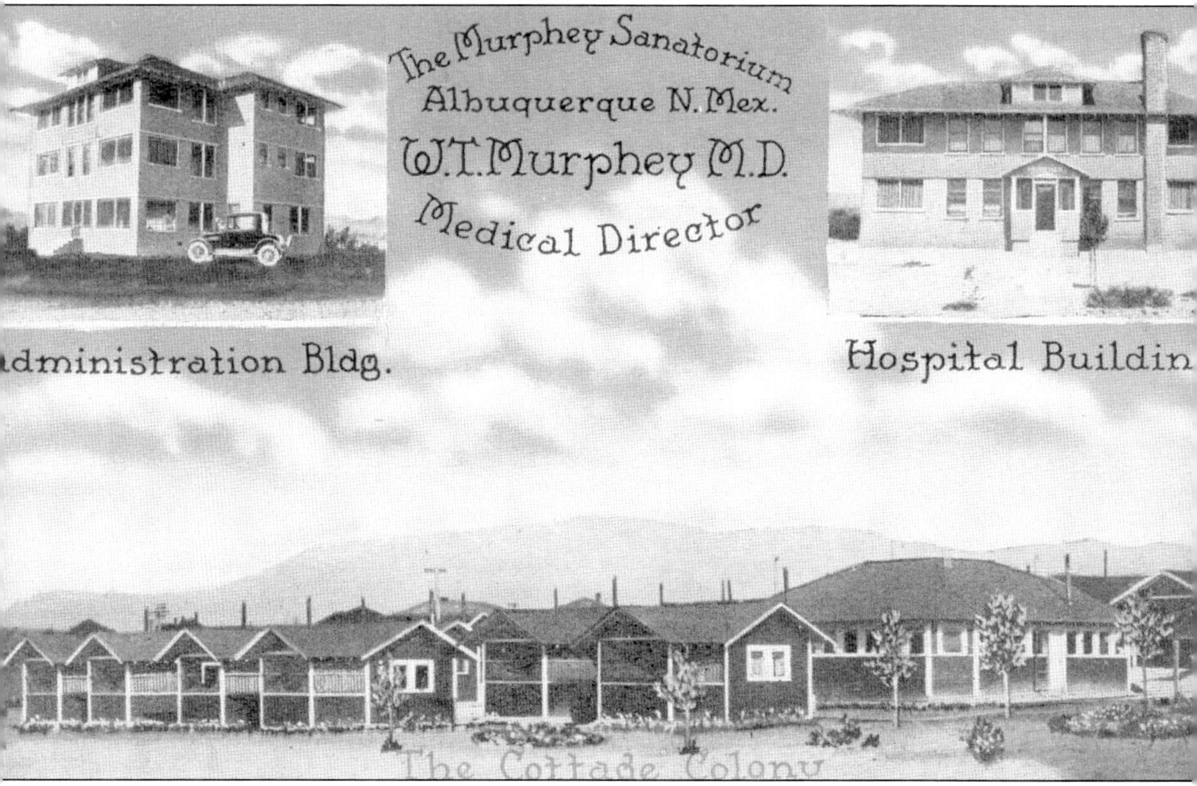

Dr. W.T. Murphey founded Albuquerque's Murphey Sanatorium in 1915. Designed in the Prairie style, the Murphey san was the last cottage san to be built in Albuquerque. Like other doctors who operated their own sans, Dr. Murphey appealed directly to family doctors across the country, urging them to place their TB patients in his care. In 1919, for example, Murphey mailed this postcard as a "cordial invitation" to a doctor in Spokane, Washington, to inspect every part of the Albuquerque san. Dr. Murphey also urged the physician to "feel free" to write for "detailed particulars." (Courtesy of Nancy Tucker.)

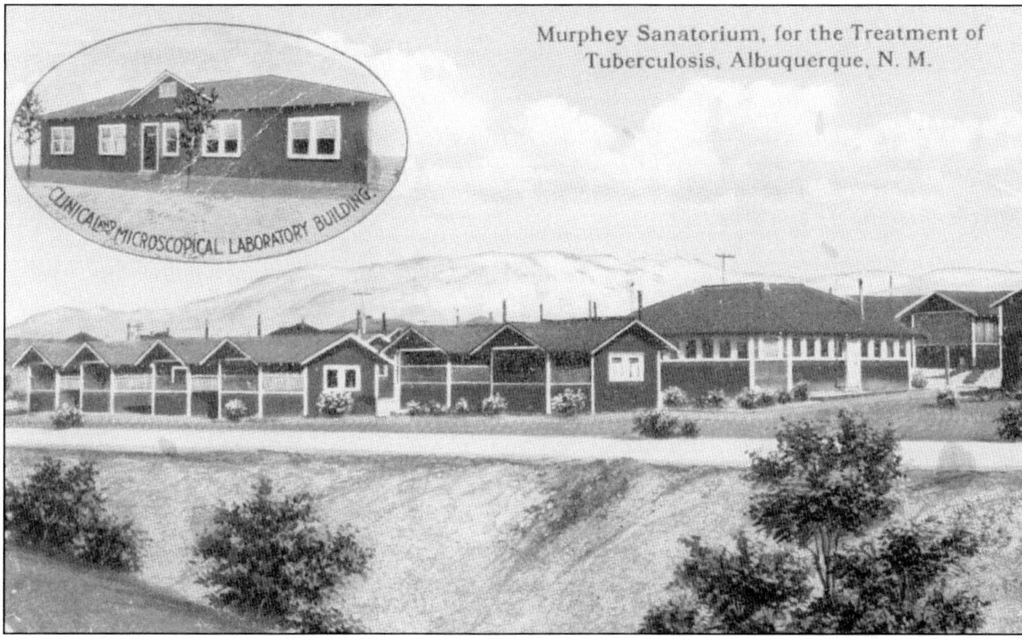

Dr. Murphey's marketing strategy met with success for at least six years, until 1921, when he sold his san to the Episcopal Church, which renamed it St. John's Sanatorium. Murphey stayed on as medical director. The san advertised to various organizations, including unions, like the Brotherhood of Locomotive Firemen and Engineers. St. John's was sold to J. Crowley in 1927. Doctors had given Crowley only 30 days to live when he first arrived in New Mexico from Butte, Montana. Defying the odds, Crowley recovered and operated his own san, ominously named the Sunset Lodge, when he bought St. John's. Renaming it the Hillcrest Sanatorium, Crowley admitted 65 patients in his first six weeks of business. By 1931, the san maxed out with 85 patients.

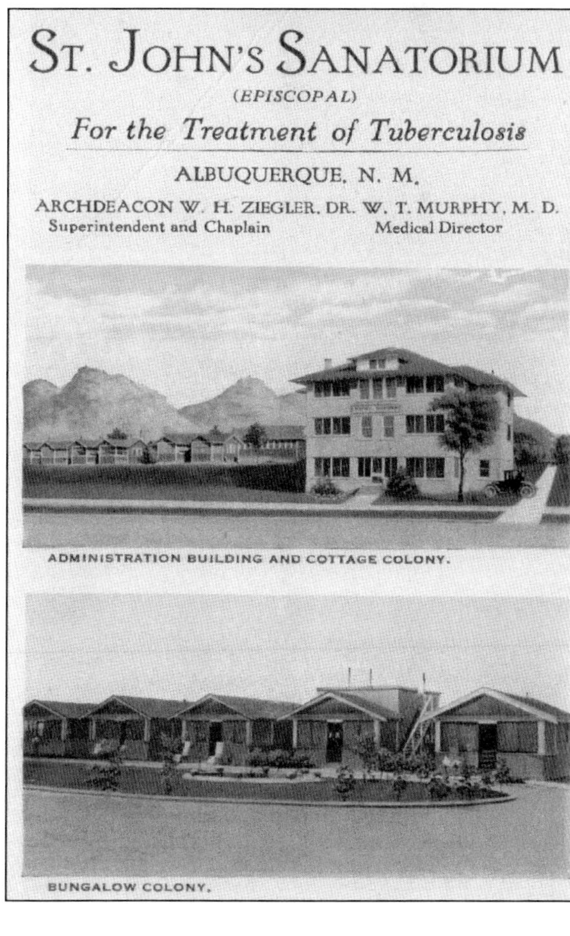

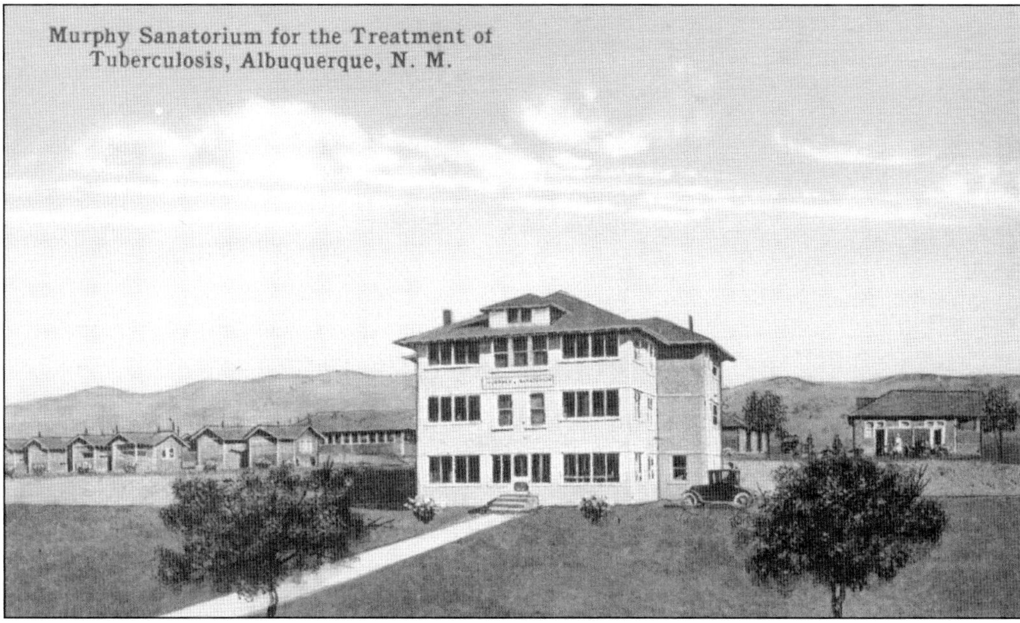
Murphy Sanatorium for the Treatment of
Tuberculosis, Albuquerque, N. M.

Conditions at Hillcrest (formerly Murphey's) Sanatorium worsened during the Great Depression. In 1934, Hillcrest's remaining 36 patients were notified that the san was closing. Hillcrest soon reopened, but its heating plant broke down in 1936, and a fire destroyed its dining room and kitchen in 1937. With inadequate insurance to cover damages, the san closed for good; its last patients scattered as far away as Deming. (Courtesy of Jim Coad.)

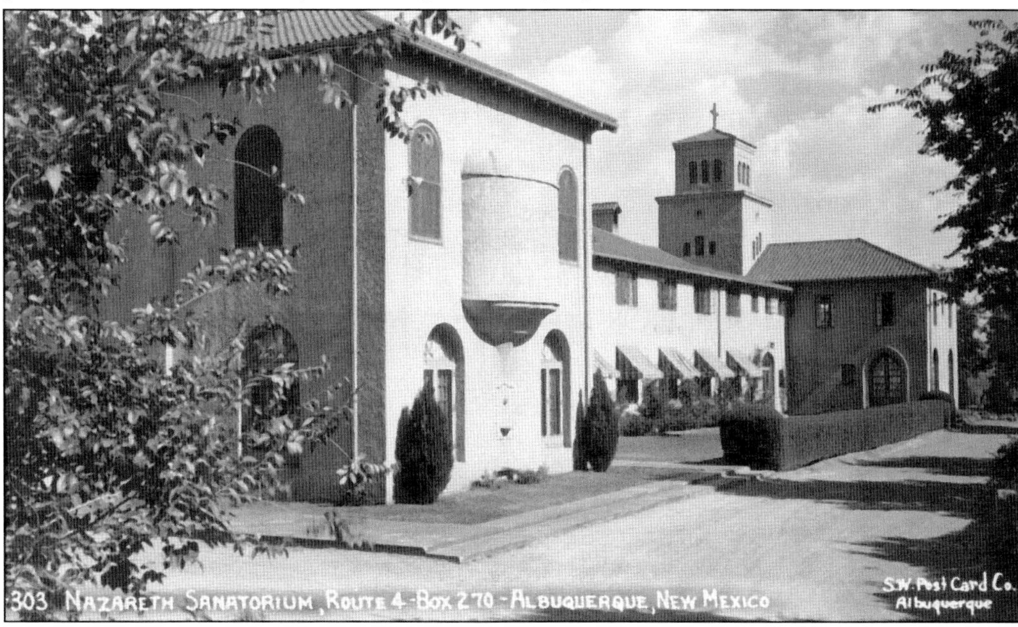
303 Nazareth Sanatorium, Route 4-Box 270 - Albuquerque, New Mexico
S.W. Post Card Co.
Albuquerque

In 1930, five sisters of the Dominican Sisters opened the 10-room Nazareth Sanatorium on Alameda Boulevard. The Dominican Sisters financed 100 percent of the cost. By 1946, the small san had been converted into an institution for patients with nervous disorders and mental illnesses. The institution faced national criticism when a 17-year-old girl underwent 62 electric shock treatments over a three-month period in 1959. (Courtesy of Nancy Tucker.)

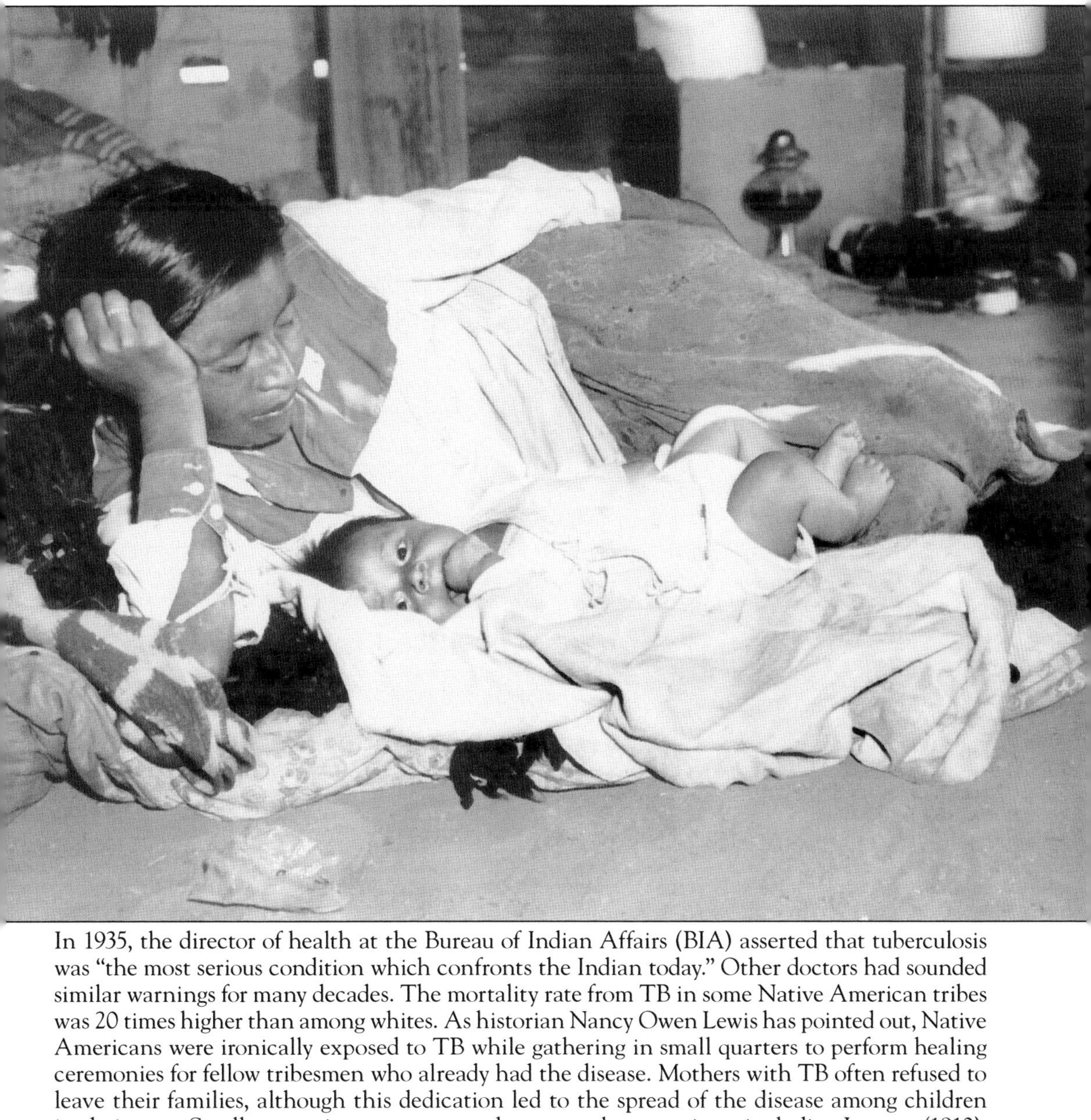

In 1935, the director of health at the Bureau of Indian Affairs (BIA) asserted that tuberculosis was "the most serious condition which confronts the Indian today." Other doctors had sounded similar warnings for many decades. The mortality rate from TB in some Native American tribes was 20 times higher than among whites. As historian Nancy Owen Lewis has pointed out, Native Americans were ironically exposed to TB while gathering in small quarters to perform healing ceremonies for fellow tribesmen who already had the disease. Mothers with TB often refused to leave their families, although this dedication led to the spread of the disease among children in their care. Small sanatoriums were opened on several reservations, including Laguna (1910), Zuni (1913), Mescalero Apache (1916), and Jicarilla Apache (1921), but the need for a larger, more modern facility continued through the 1920s.

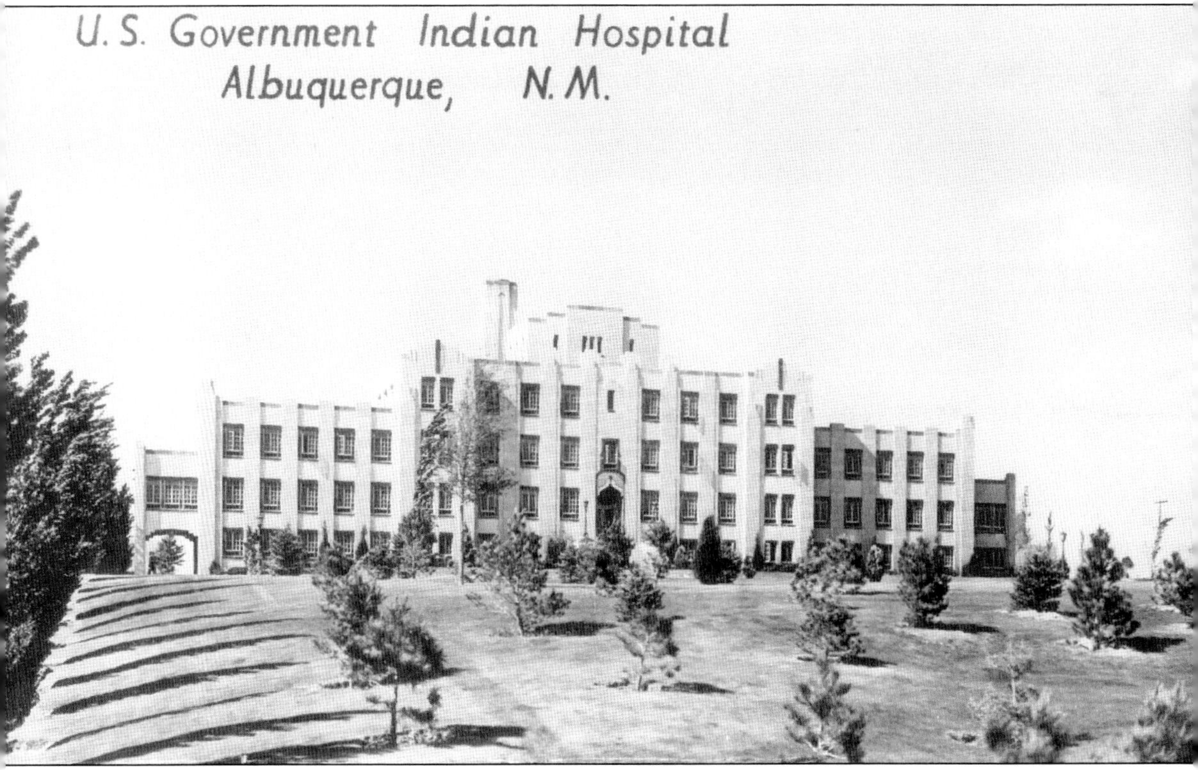

In response to the dire need for an Indian sanatorium in New Mexico, plans to build a $375,000 san were announced in 1931. Designed by BIA architect Hans Stamm in the Pueblo Deco style, the building was the first BIA structure that deviated from the bureau's standard institutional designs. Interior walls, tiles, and ceilings were decorated with Indian motifs. An arrow motif appeared on the high smokestack to the rear of the four-story, symmetrical building. Rejecting the old cottage plan, the new facility cared for its patients in one large building. The san was so isolated on an unpaved road (now Lomas Boulevard) that a cattle guard had to be built to prevent cattle from grazing on its landscaped grounds. (Courtesy of Nancy Tucker.)

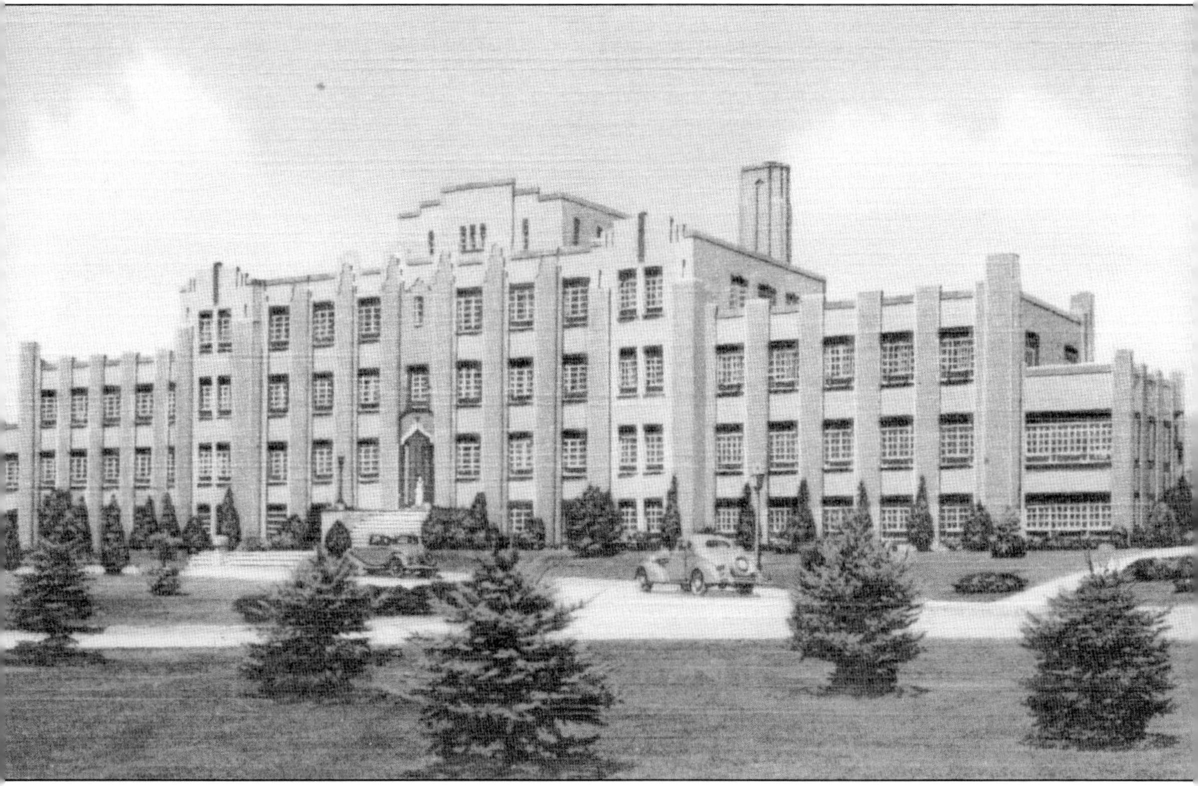

With so many Native Americans afflicted with TB, the Indian Sanatorium's 110 available beds were full from the start. Almost 900 patients were admitted in the first six years alone. Patients came from tribes across the United States; translators were often required to communicate with the non-Indian staff. Patients' ages ranged from children to a man who said he was 108. Patients stayed for an average of one year; there was no charge for their care. The TB crisis among Native Americans continued into the 1950s and 1960s; a fourth of all deaths from TB in New Mexico in 1951 were Native Americans. As a result, the US Public Health Service (PHS) signed a contract with Presbyterian Hospital and the Fort Stanton Tuberculosis Hospital to care for Navajo patients who could not be admitted to the consistently full Albuquerque Indian Sanatorium.

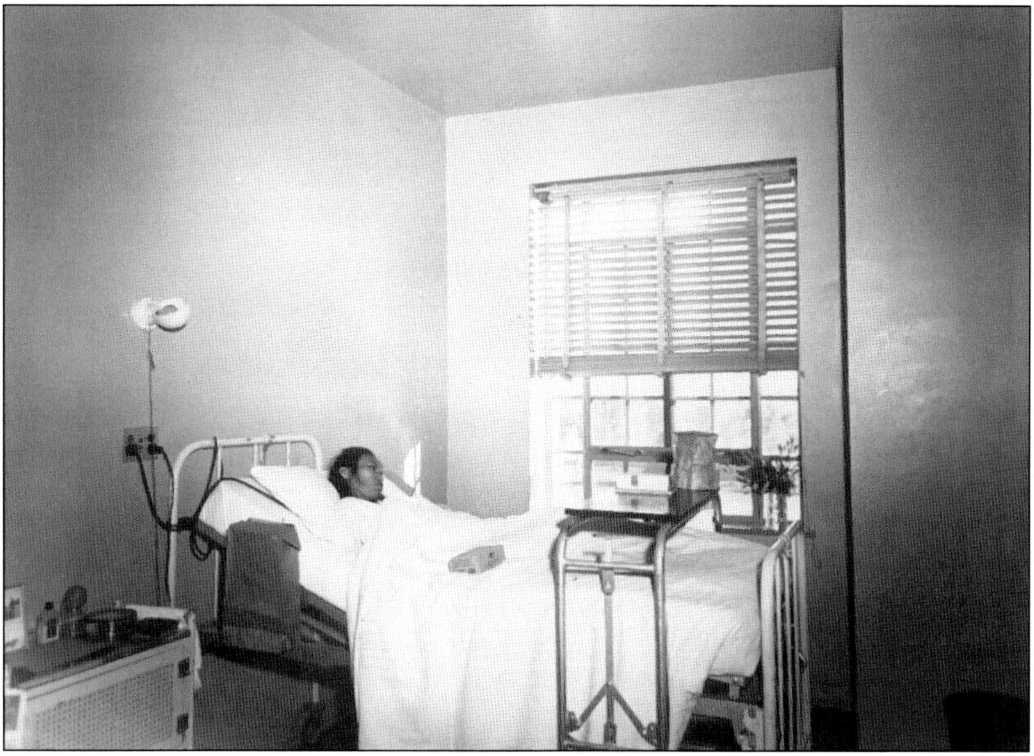

Like every san that has survived, the Indian san eventually expanded to become a general hospital. The need for such an institution was so great that a $16 million addition was built in 1982. The addition caused an uproar among historic preservationists, because it upstaged the original structure, physically and in terms of design. By 1995, the hospital served over 30,000 patients per year. Overall, it had served members of 222 different tribes in the course of its long history.

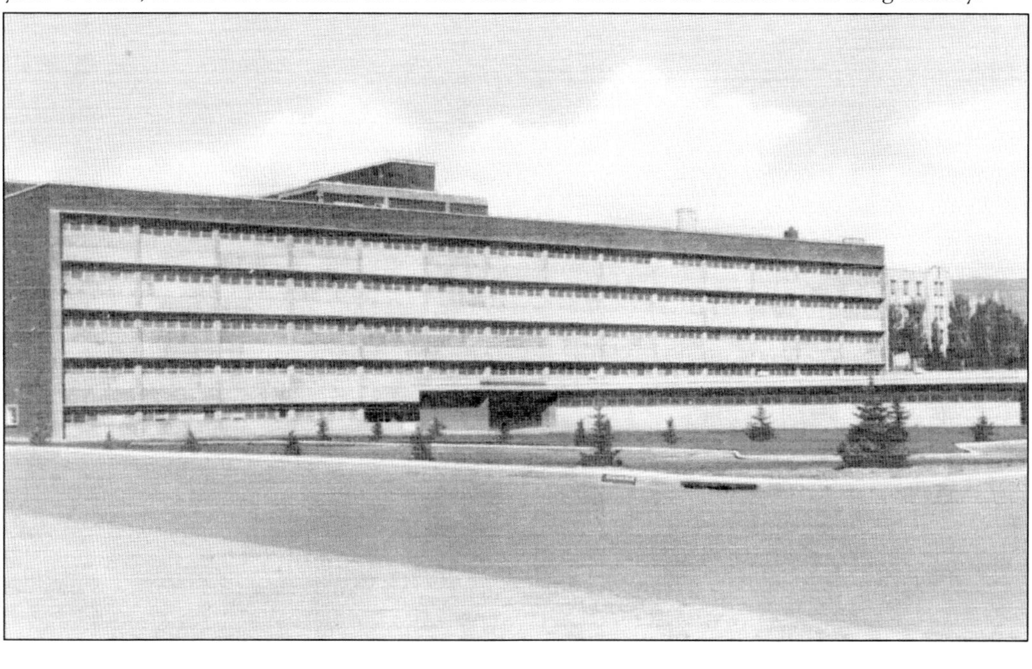

Six

New Mexico's Military Sanatoriums

Every segment of American society suffered the ravages of tuberculosis. The military was no exception. The number of veterans with TB reached crisis proportions after the Spanish-American War and World War I. The US Soldiers Home in Washington, DC, could not handle the enormous burden.

A firm believer in climate therapy, Surgeon General of the Army George M. Sternberg identified Fort Bayard as an ideal location for the military's first sanatorium to treat veterans plagued with TB. Buffalo soldiers had helped establish the fort in 1866. It had been named for Brig. Gen. George Bayard, who had been killed in combat during the Civil War.

Closed with the end of the Indian wars, the fort reopened as a TB sanatorium in 1899. The facility remained an Army hospital until 1920, when the US Public Health Service took charge. A new hospital was built in 1922, when operations were transferred to the Veterans' Bureau. In 1965, the VA transferred ownership to the state of New Mexico, which used the property as a long-term health-care facility. A new Fort Bayard Medical Center was opened in 2010. With 400 beds, Fort Bayard was once the largest san in New Mexico and the largest government facility of its kind in the country.

Fort Stanton in Lincoln County was also chosen as the location for a new government sanatorium, but for members of the merchant marines rather than for Army veterans. Established in 1855, the fort was named after Capt. Henry W. Stanton, who had been killed in an Indian ambush. Like Fort Bayard, the military installation had been decommissioned in 1896, but, three years later, had been chosen as the site of the Fort Stanton Marine Hospital. Second in capacity only to Fort Bayard in New Mexico, Fort Stanton grew to serve an estimated 5,000 merchant marines from 1899 to 1953. In 1953, it was transferred to the State of New Mexico to serve as a TB hospital. Closed in 1966, Fort Stanton has, in the succeeding years, served many functions, from a women's prison to a drug and alcohol rehabilitation center.

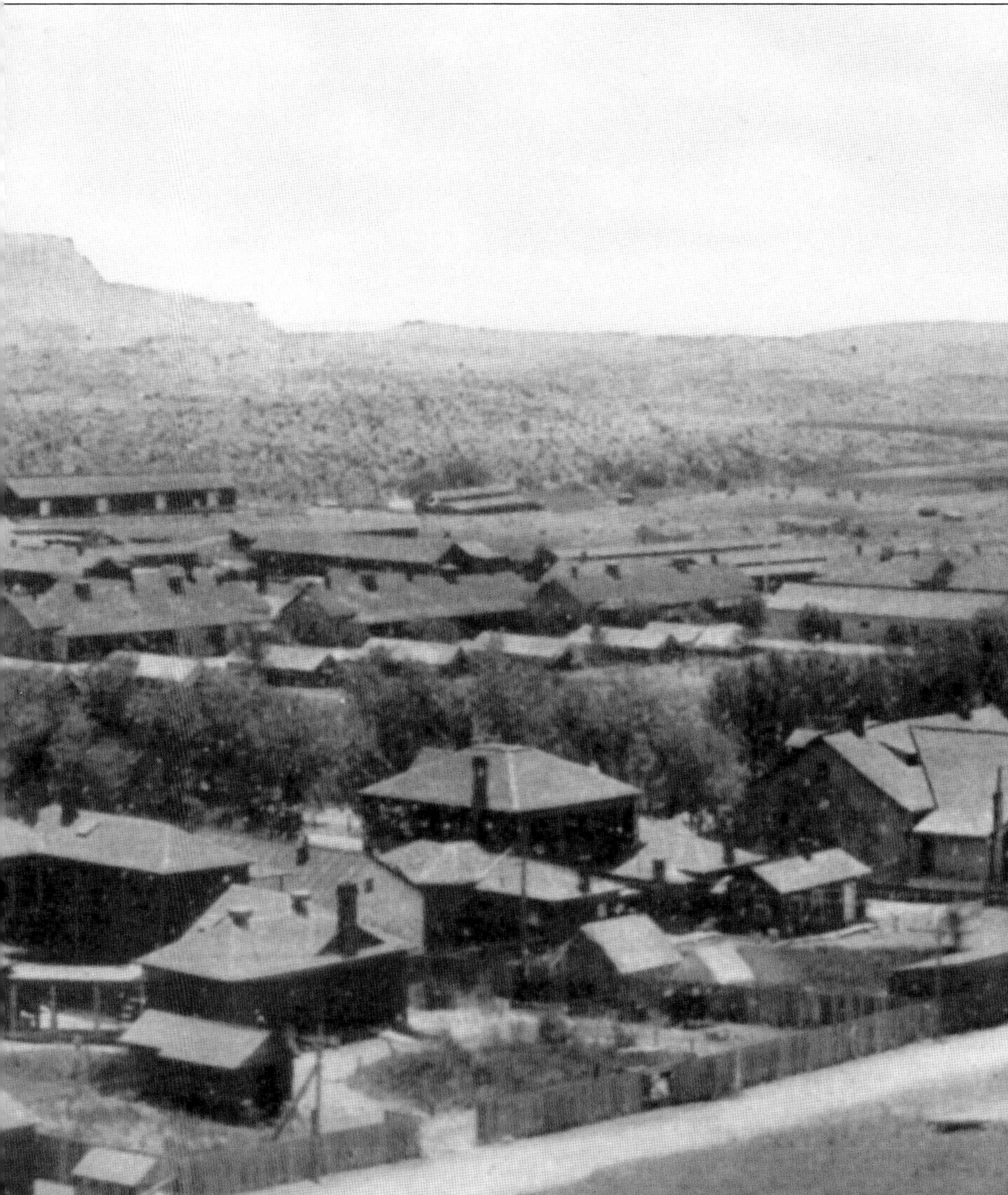

A 1900 *Albuquerque Journal* article notes how "scrupulously clean" everything was kept at Fort Bayard, including all of the patients; the men were required to "bathe at least once each week." Patients were also required to make their own beds, keep their belongings "neatly arranged," and

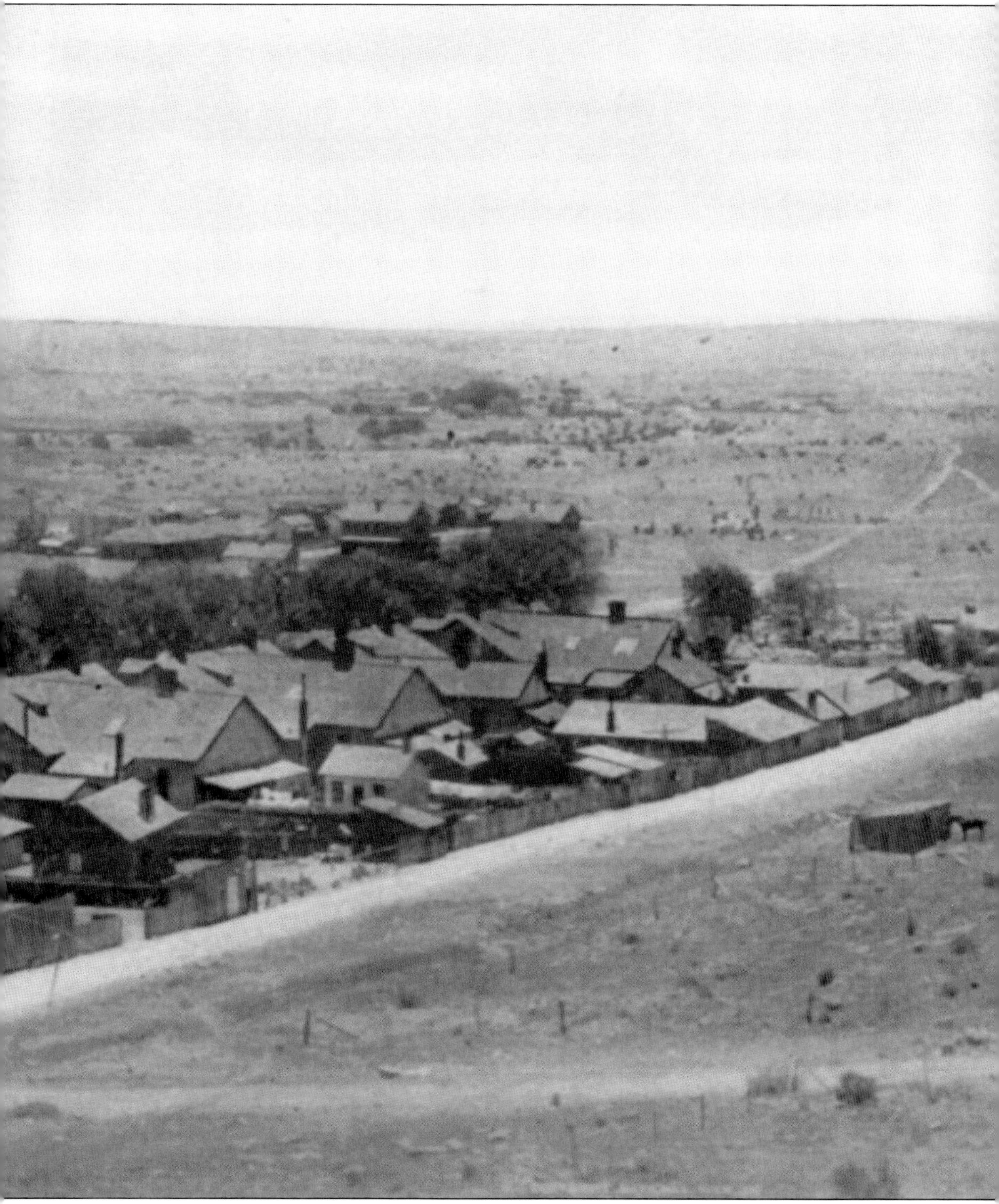

make sure that their whiskers and mustaches were "kept closely trimmed." Of most importance, patients were expected to spit in provided paper cups, which had to be burned when half full or every 24 hours, whichever came first. (Courtesy of Nancy Tucker.)

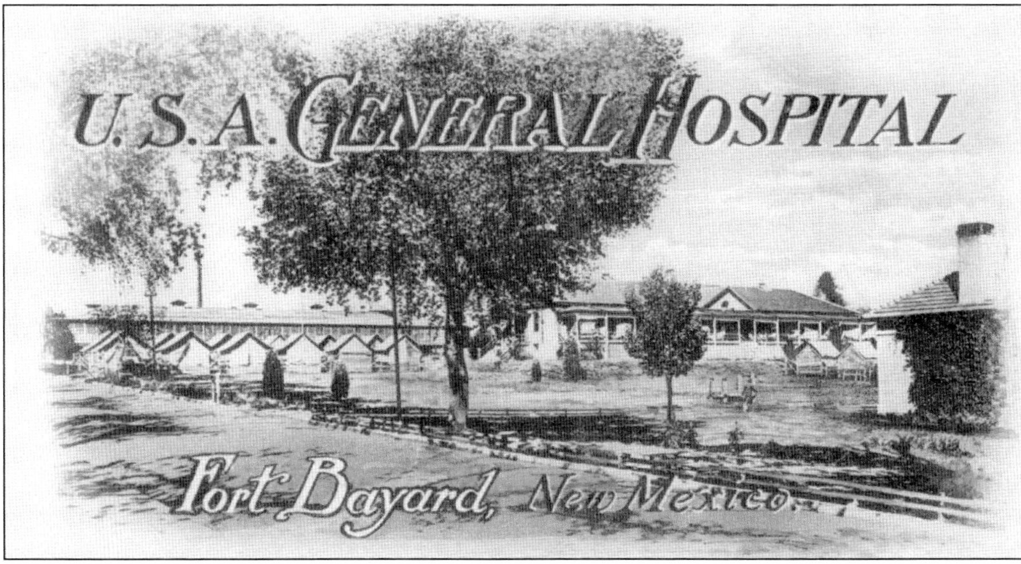

Unlike private sans, Fort Bayard had no need to market its services with slick promotional brochures and postcards. It nevertheless produced attractive postcards as a convenient means for patients to write short notes reassuring loved ones of their well-being. (Courtesy of Nancy Tucker.)

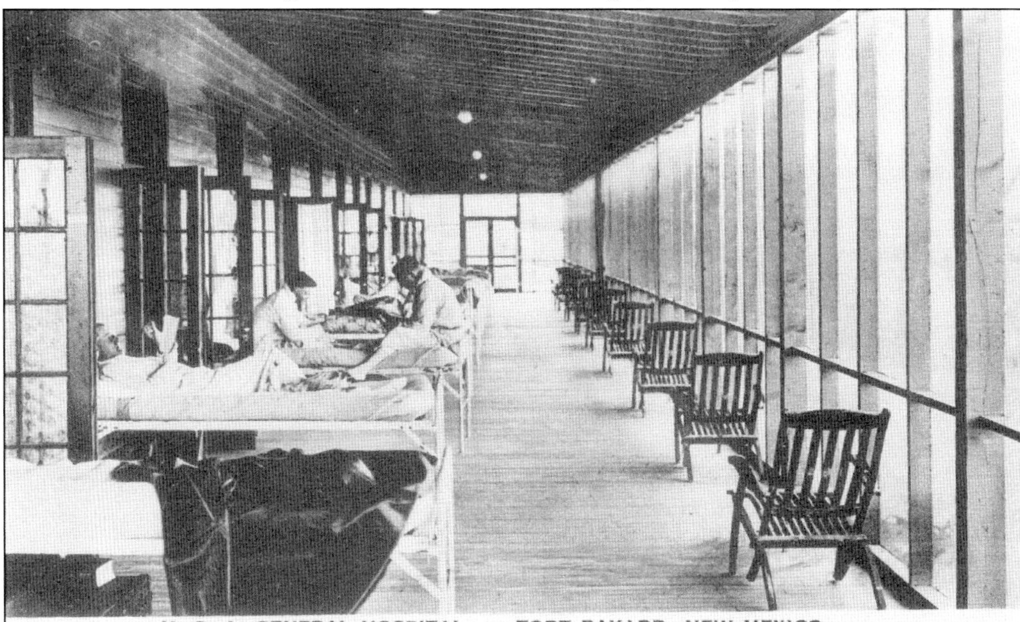

To receive the maximum amount of fresh air, patients could not occupy their quarters between 8:00 a.m. and 7:30 p.m.; they were strongly urged to remain outdoors at least eight hours daily. Patients were required to sleep on verandas in all seasons. Calling their buildings "ships," men survived cold weather by wearing woolen hats and heavy sheepskin coats while covering themselves with oiled canvas blankets. Hospital patients wore pajamas during most hours of the day and night. Patients could pick up a change of clean pajamas daily from the central supply room. Patients in the 1940s later remembered that men who were considered very sick were given red pajamas, while those who were in recovery were given white (some say blue) pajamas. (Courtesy of Nancy Tucker.)

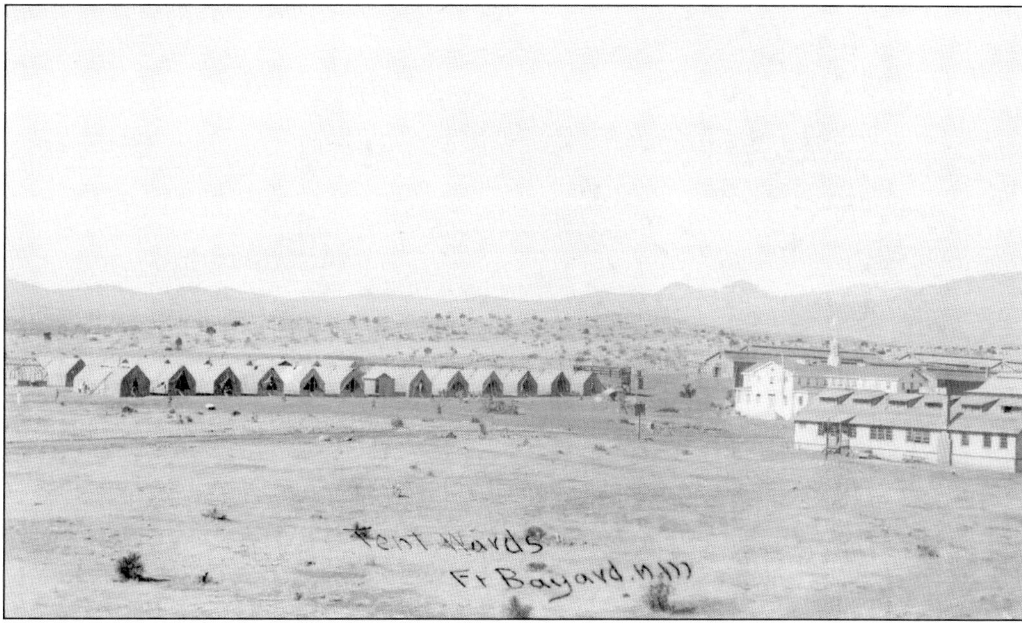
Tent Wards
Ft Bayard N.M.

Many ambulatory patients lived in tent structures, with three hospital tents placed end-to-end to provide enough space to accommodate a dozen beds in each outdoor ward. With their ongoing emphasis on breathing clean air, medical officers insisted that at least one side of each tent remain open in all but "very stormy weather." (Above, courtesy of Jim Coad; below, courtesy of Nancy Tucker.)

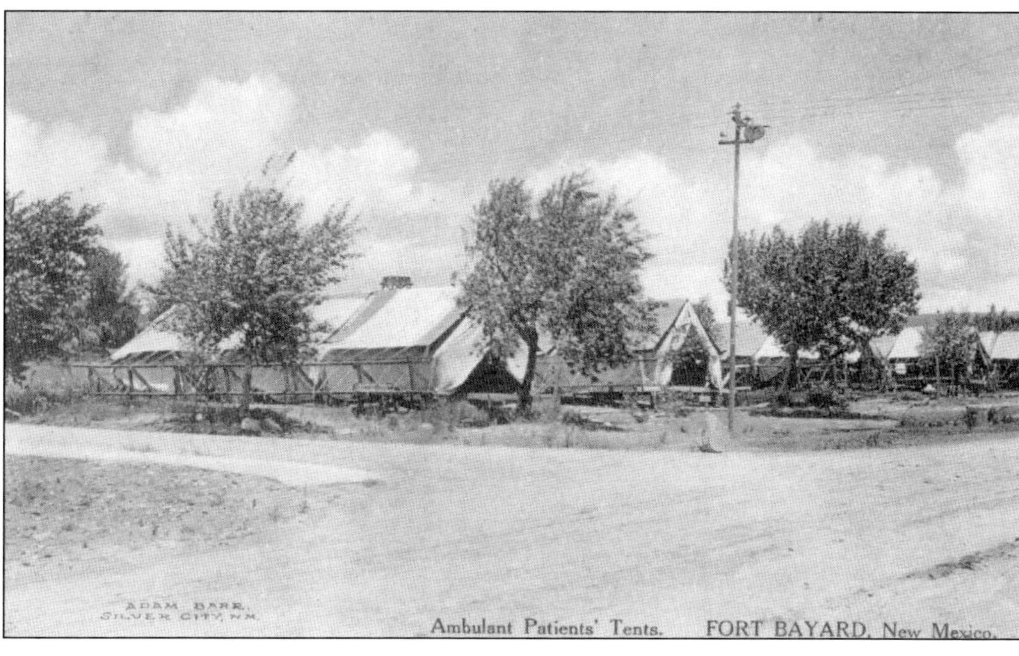
Ambulant Patients' Tents. FORT BAYARD, New Mexico.

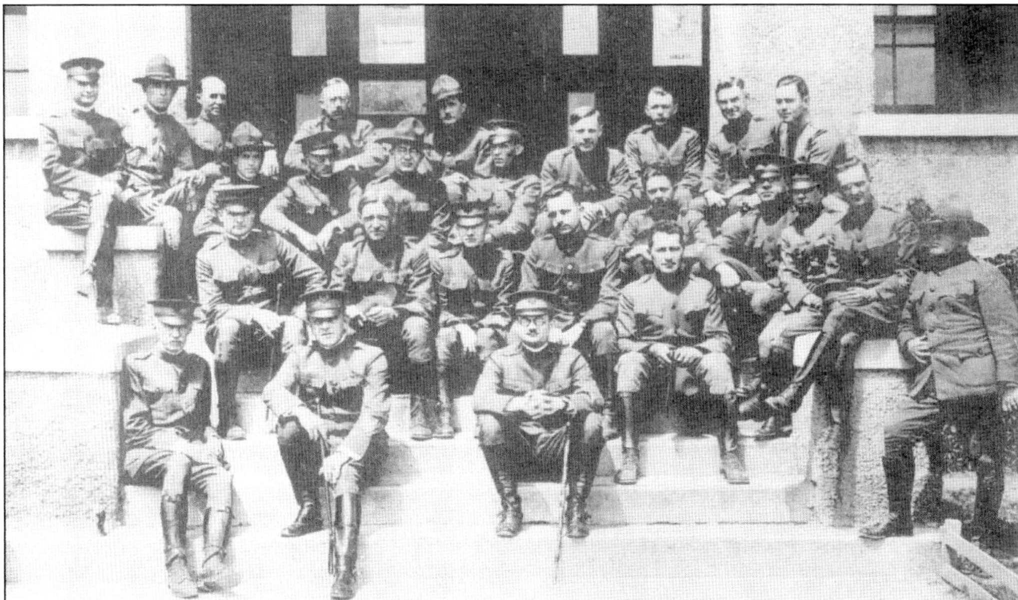

U. S. A. GENERAL HOSPITAL. FORT BAYARD. NEW MEXICO.
The Doctors who take care of us.

Fort Bayard was fortunate to have many exceptional physicians and nurses assigned to its staff. Dita Kinney served as the fort's chief nurse before her appointment as the first superintendent of the Army Nurse Corps. Maj. D.M. Appel, Dr. Earl Bullock, and Col. George Bushnell used their years at the fort to conduct valuable medical research, published in prestigious periodicals like the *Journal of the American Medical Association.* Although several of the doctors at the fort had had TB themselves, they did not always have the highest regard for patients in their care. In 1909, one physician wrote that "without a doubt no other institutions, outside those of a penal character, or insane asylums, can show quite so inferior a class of patients: equally improvident, thoughtless, dissipated, ungrateful, and to a great extent syphilized [sic]." (Both, courtesy of Nancy Tucker.)

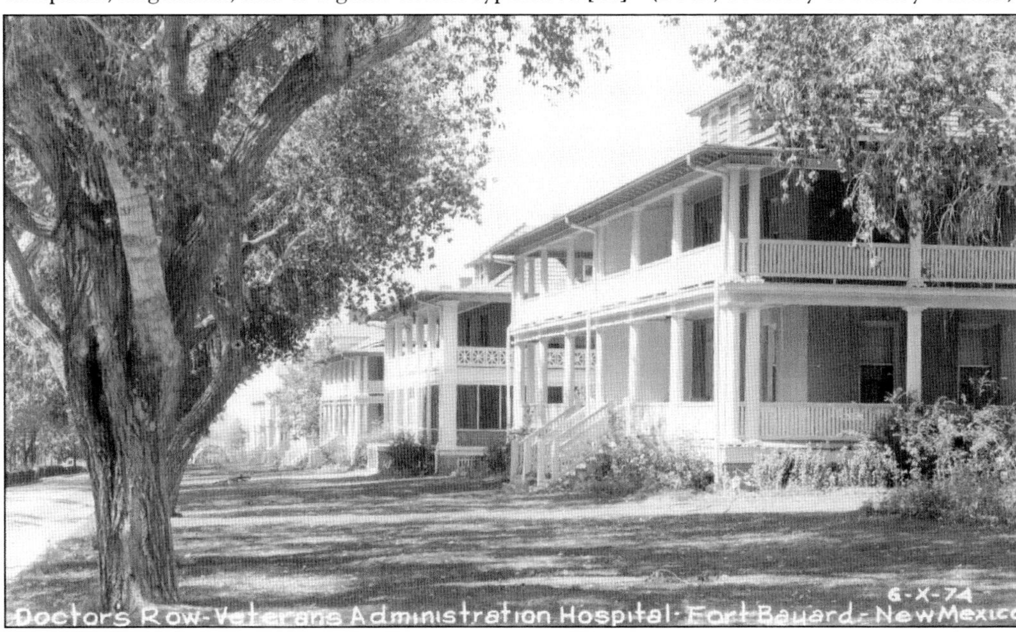
6-X-74
Doctor's Row-Veterans Administration Hospital-Fort Bayard-New Mexico

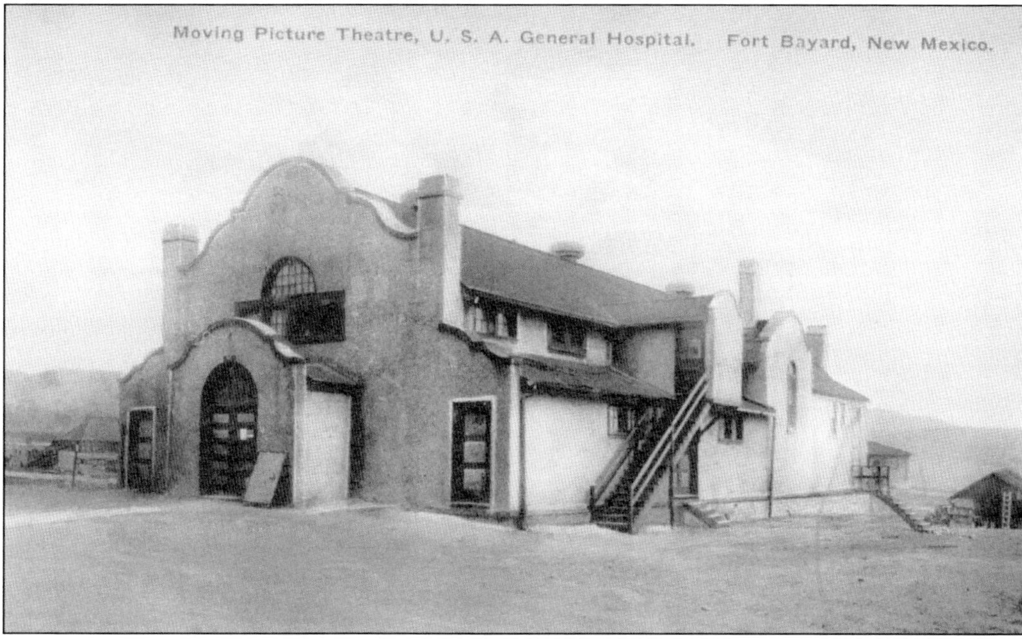

Built on the corner of the fort's old parade grounds, the amusement hall was large enough to seat 150 men at each performance. Orchestras, made up of patients and military personnel, often performed at the hall, as did traveling acting companies and lecturers who used lantern slides to illustrate their presentations. Vaudeville shows by "members of the garrison" were popular as well. Movies, including talkies, were shown by the 1930s. (Both, courtesy of Nancy Tucker.)

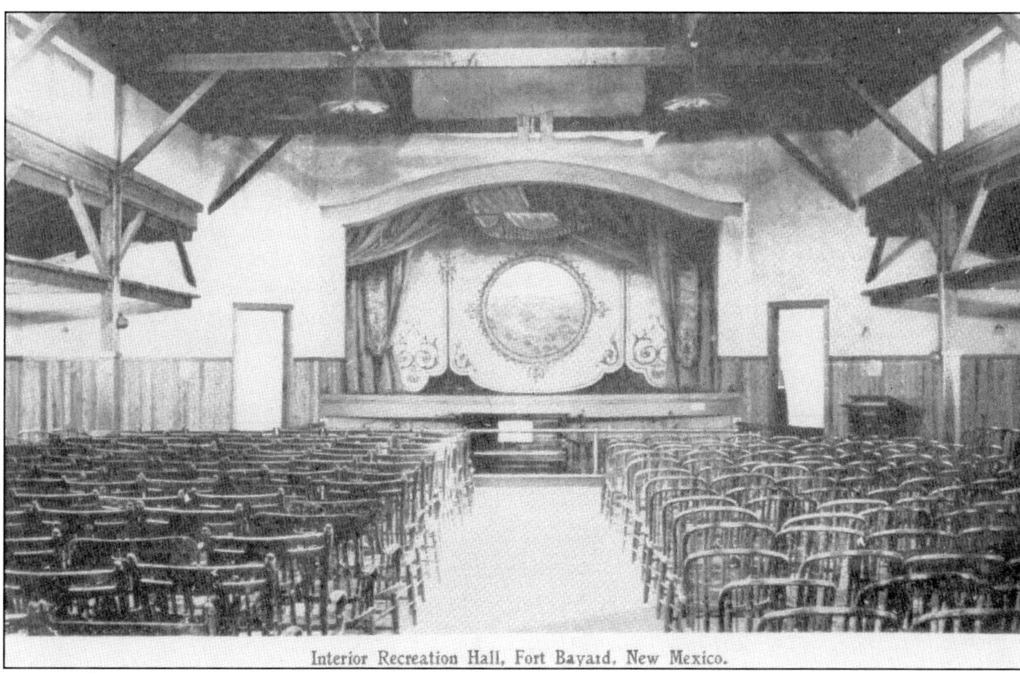

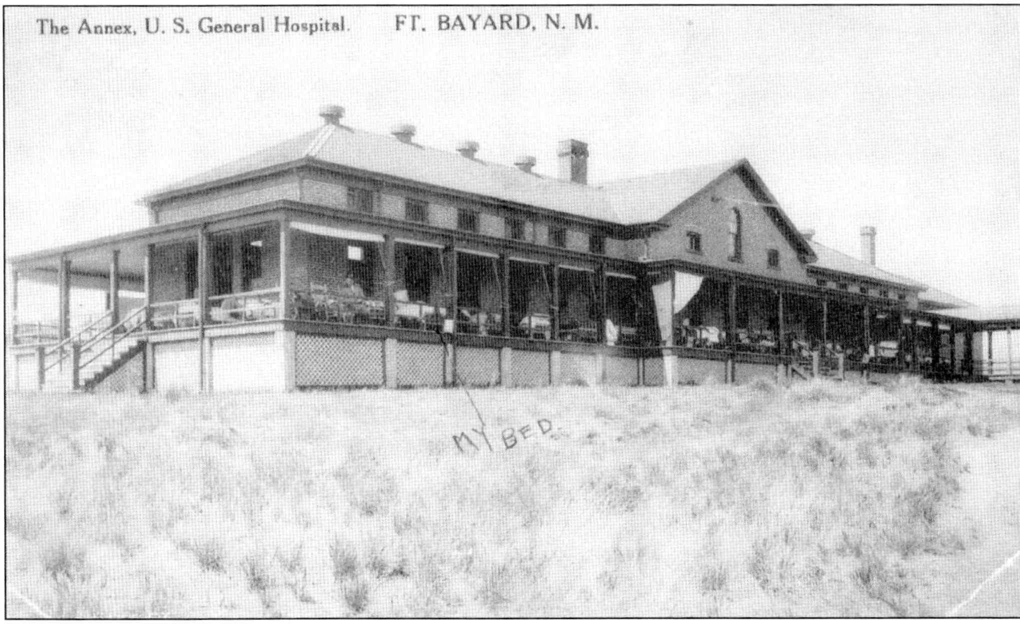

After World War I, when rumors spread that Fort Bayard was about to become a veterans hospital, many patients objected, insisting that veterans would be better served if the new VA hospital was located elsewhere. Assisted by the new American Legion, disgruntled patients met at a mass meeting in August 1921. They complained that the fort was too far from the nearest train depot; that the stores in Silver City were too expensive; and that at least three old wards should be demolished. Despite these protests, the federal government decided to build several new structures and open its newest VA hospital at Fort Bayard. The facility opened on May 1, 1922, with Gen. "Black Jack" Pershing, who had served at the fort in 1886, in attendance as an honored guest. (Both, courtesy of Nancy Tucker.)

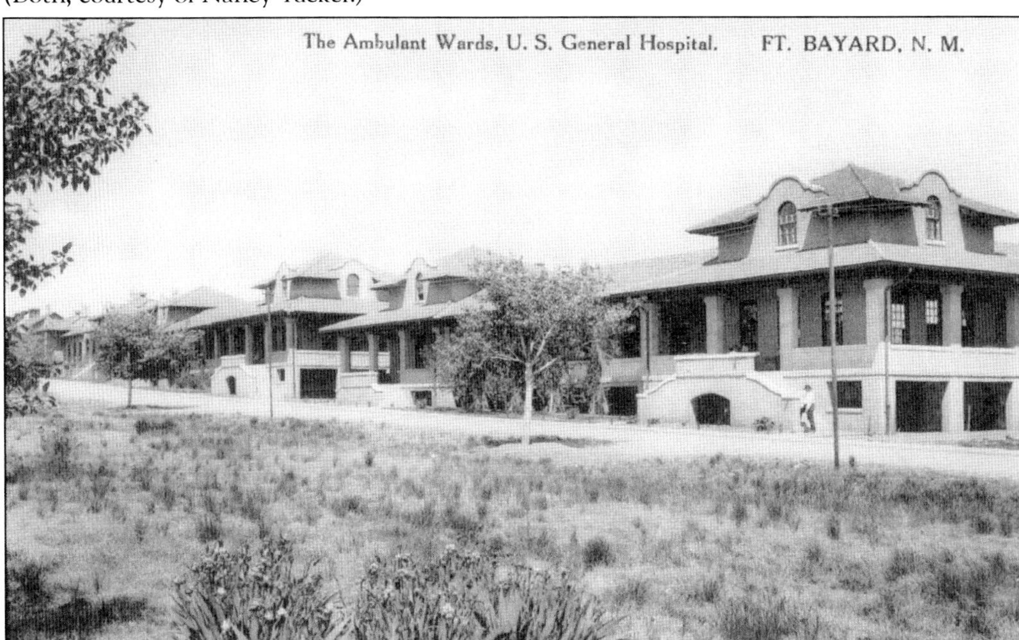

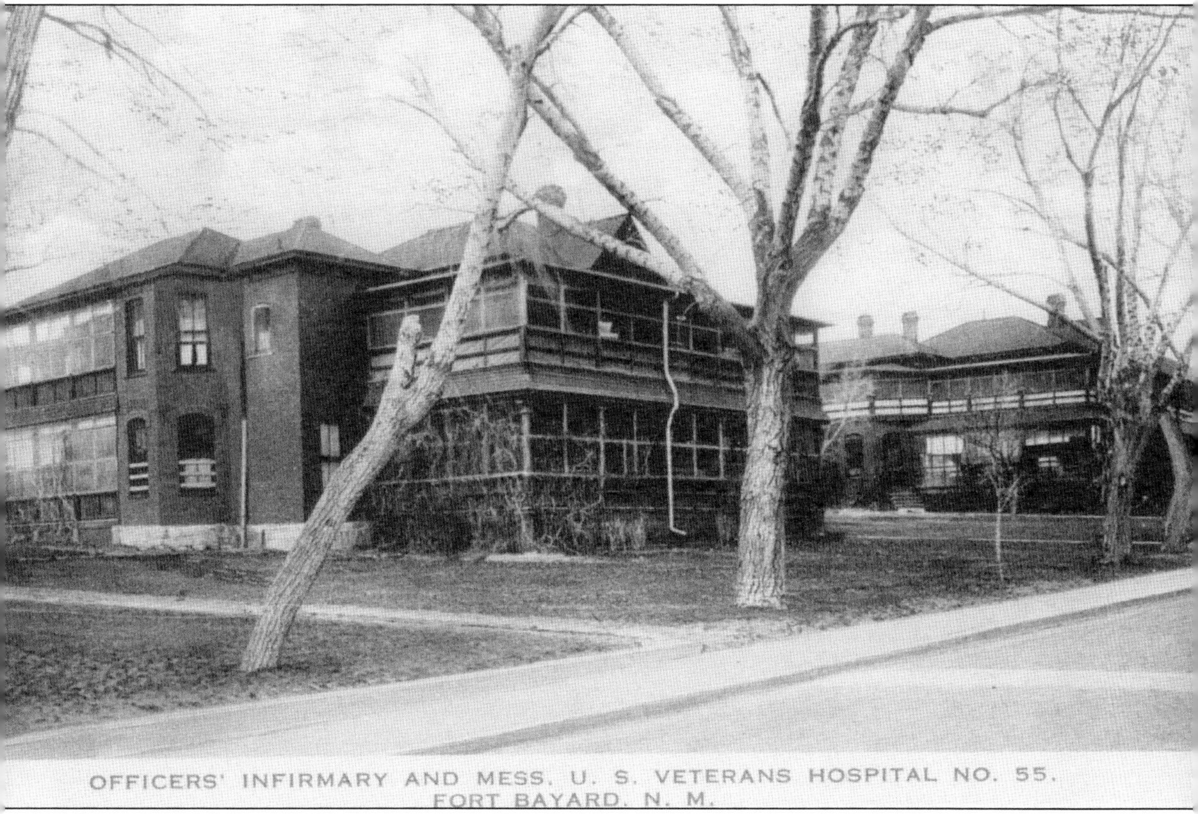

The onset of the Great Depression brought new fears to Fort Bayard, as the federal government threatened to cut VA hospitals and benefits across the country. In mid-1933, rumors spread that Fort Bayard would be among the hospitals to be closed, because it was considered too isolated. Sen. Bronson Cutting, a veteran and former lunger himself, visited the fort to listen to the patients' concerns. Cutting's influence may well have saved Fort Bayard from closing at the height of the nation's economic disaster. Rather than closing, the fort benefited from a series of landscape and construction projects under New Deal programs like the Works Progress Administration (WPA) and the Civilian Conservation Corps (CCC). (Courtesy of Nancy Tucker.)

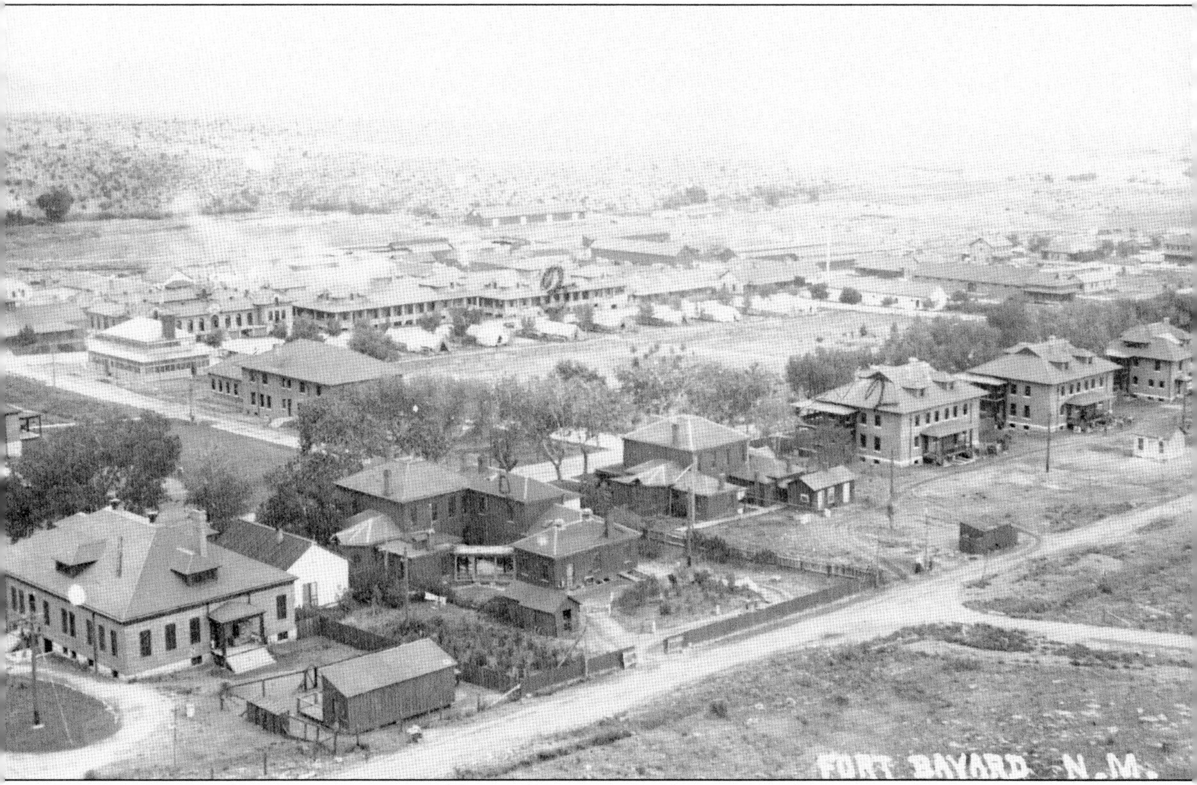

Fort Bayard began to receive additional patients in late December 1941, when West Coast VA hospitals transferred 110 patients to make room for anticipated casualties during World War II. Many military doctors and nurses were transferred to fronts in Europe and the Pacific. Maintenance personnel also joined the military. With the shortage of workers, about 100 prisoners from the German POW camp in Lordsburg were brought to Fort Bayard in 1944 to serve as orderlies and groundskeepers. Those who knew these Germans described them as "the nicest bunch of people you could ever hope to know." (Courtesy of Nancy Tucker.)

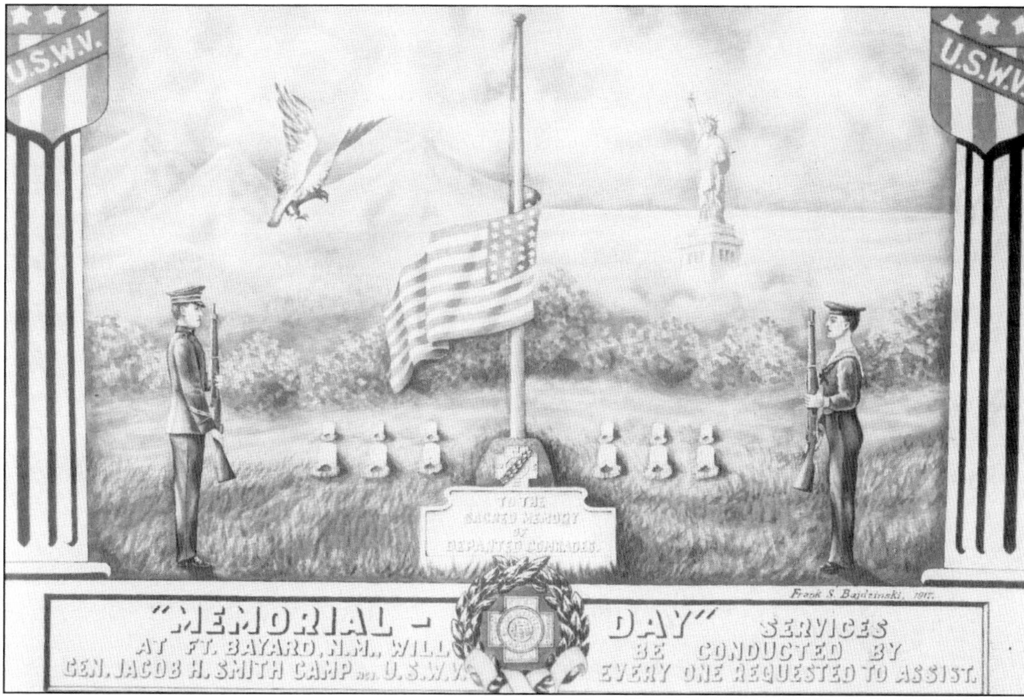
U.S.W.V.
U.S.W.V.
TO THE SACRED MEMORY OF DEPARTED COMRADES.
"MEMORIAL - DAY" SERVICES
AT FT. BAYARD, N.M., WILL BE CONDUCTED BY
GEN. JACOB H. SMITH CAMP U.S.W.V. EVERY ONE REQUESTED TO ASSIST.

Fort Bayard's military cemetery dates to the fort's establishment in 1866. Hundreds of patients who failed to recover from TB are buried there, as are many other veterans. New patients complained that the first place they saw when they entered the fort was its cemetery, hardly a good way to begin their fights against TB. The burial grounds became a national cemetery in 1976. (Courtesy of Nancy Tucker.)

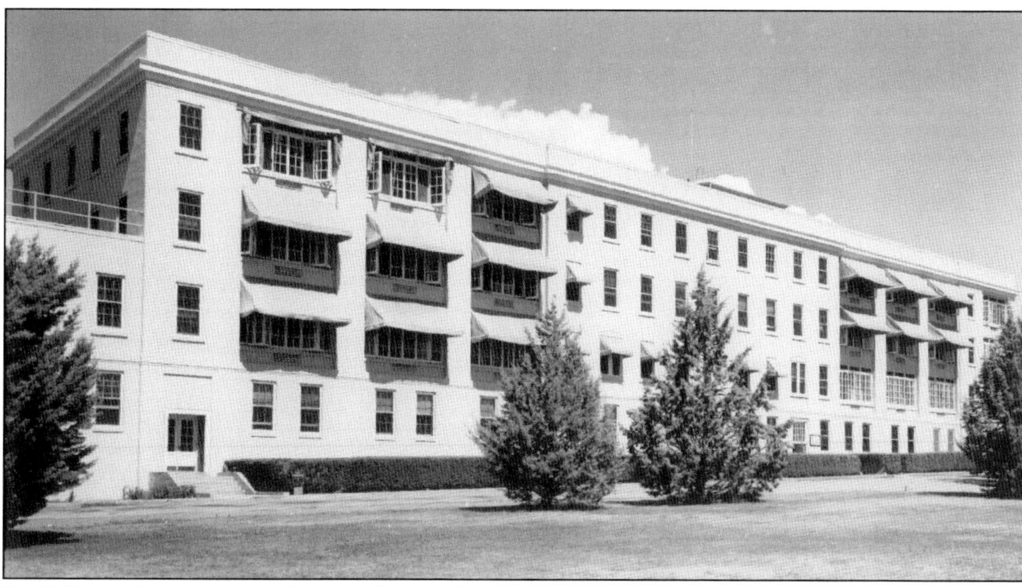

In 1965, the VA transferred ownership to the State of New Mexico, which used the property as a long-term care facility. A new 200-bed Fort Bayard Medical Center was opened in 2010. Despite the work of preservationists like Cecilia Bell, and the fort's status as a National Historic Landmark, its closing and demolition are constant threats. (Courtesy of Nancy Tucker.)

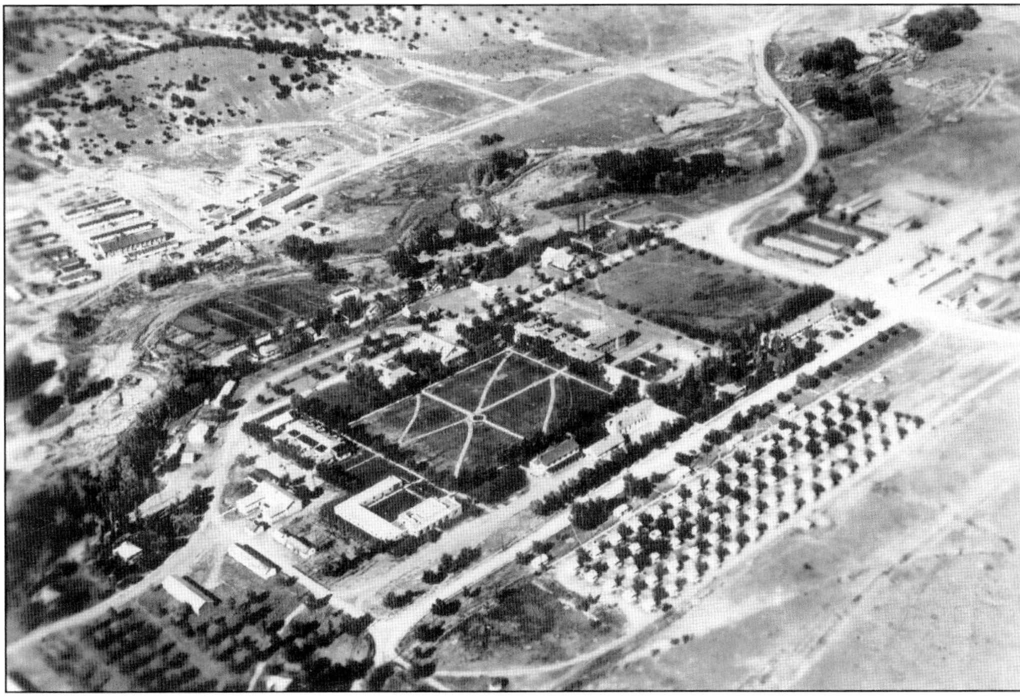

To qualify for admission to the ironically landlocked US Marine Hospital No. 9 of the US Public Health Service, a TB patient had to have served for at least three months on a merchant marine vessel flying the American flag. Joseph Ryan was the first patient admitted, in November 1899. Dr. J.O. Cobb served as the hospital's first medical director. (Courtesy of Jim Coad.)

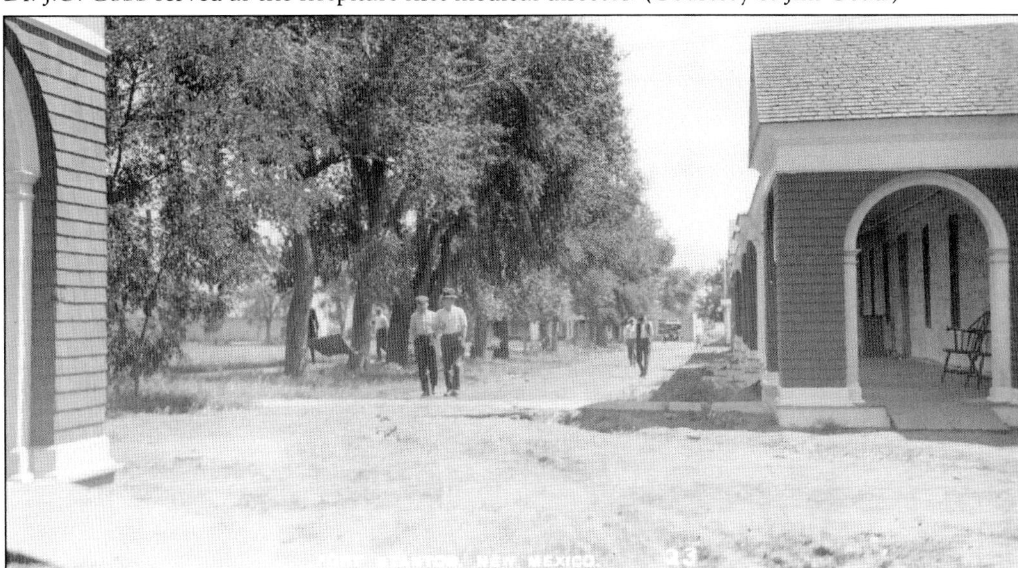

Reflecting the military fort it once was, Fort Stanton's regulations seemed endless. Patients needed passes to leave the "reservation." No one could own firearms or cars without permission; those with firearms could not discharge them within a mile of the fort. Patients could not own pets without permission; pets without metal tags could be "humanely destroyed." Patients were allowed to smoke, although it was not encouraged. (Courtesy of Nancy Tucker.)

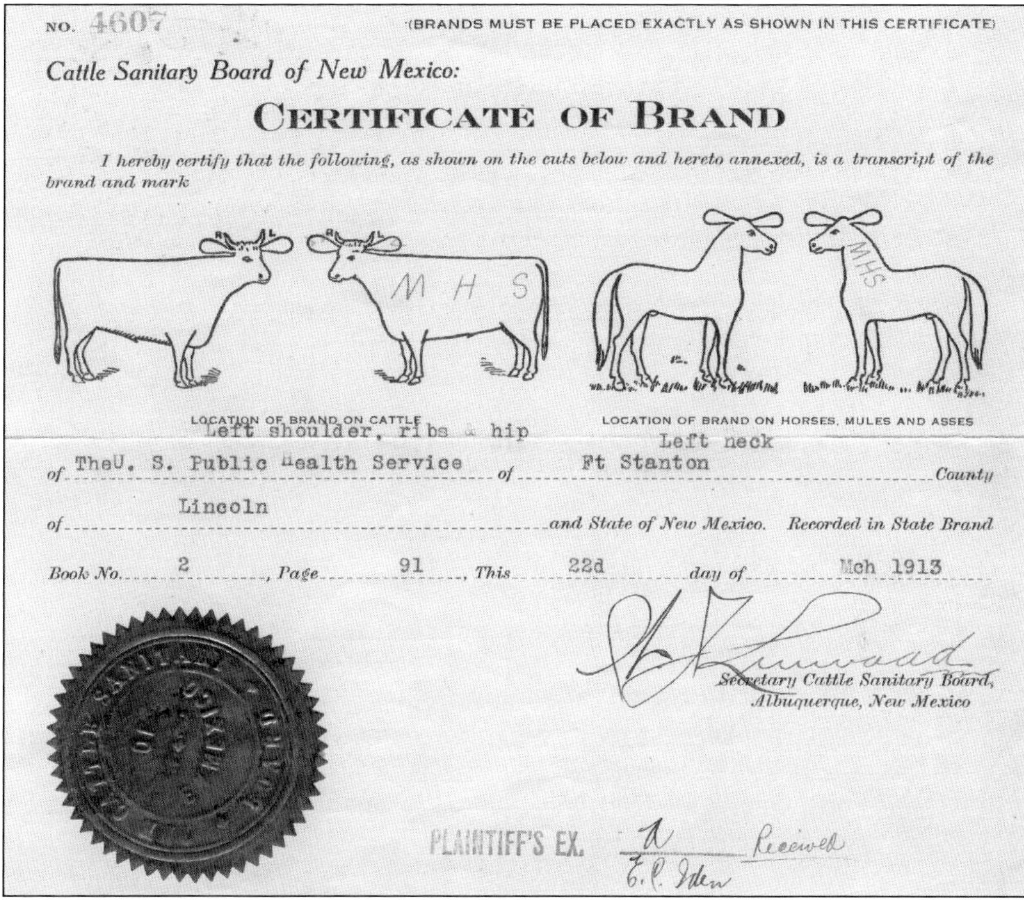

NO. 4607 (BRANDS MUST BE PLACED EXACTLY AS SHOWN IN THIS CERTIFICATE)

Cattle Sanitary Board of New Mexico:

CERTIFICATE OF BRAND

I hereby certify that the following, as shown on the cuts below and hereto annexed, is a transcript of the brand and mark

M H S

MHS

LOCATION OF BRAND ON CATTLE Left shoulder, ribs & hip

LOCATION OF BRAND ON HORSES, MULES AND ASSES Left neck

of The U. S. Public Health Service *of* Ft Stanton *County*

of Lincoln *and State of New Mexico. Recorded in State Brand*

Book No. 2, *Page* 91, *This* 22d *day of* Mch 1913

Secretary Cattle Sanitary Board, Albuquerque, New Mexico

PLAINTIFF'S EX. A Received

Public Health Service officers attempted to make Fort Stanton as self-sufficient as possible, raising 1,600 head of cattle, 50 cows (producing 100 gallons of milk a day), 200 pigs, and 500 chickens and turkeys, according to a 1908 report. Fort Stanton's cattle herd grew so large that surplus cattle were sent to other PHS hospitals in the West. In the Wild West tradition, the fort even experienced cases of cattle rustling, as happened in September 1937. For many years, Fort Stanton staged a large Fourth of July celebration, popular with residents throughout Lincoln County. The festivities included a baseball game, a barbecue, and a rodeo with horse racing, rope throwing, and wild cow milking. (Both, courtesy of Donna Henderson.)

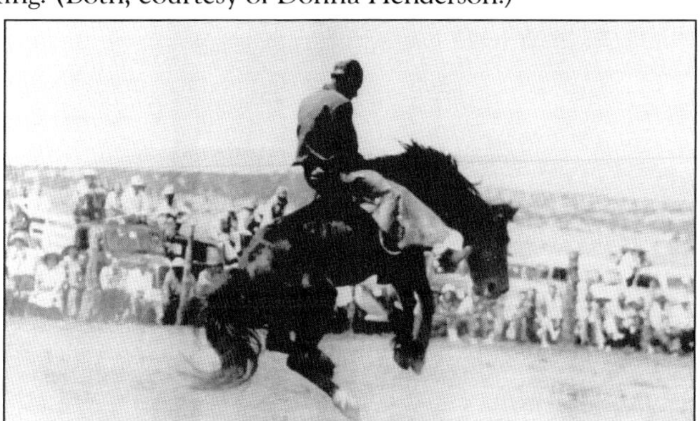

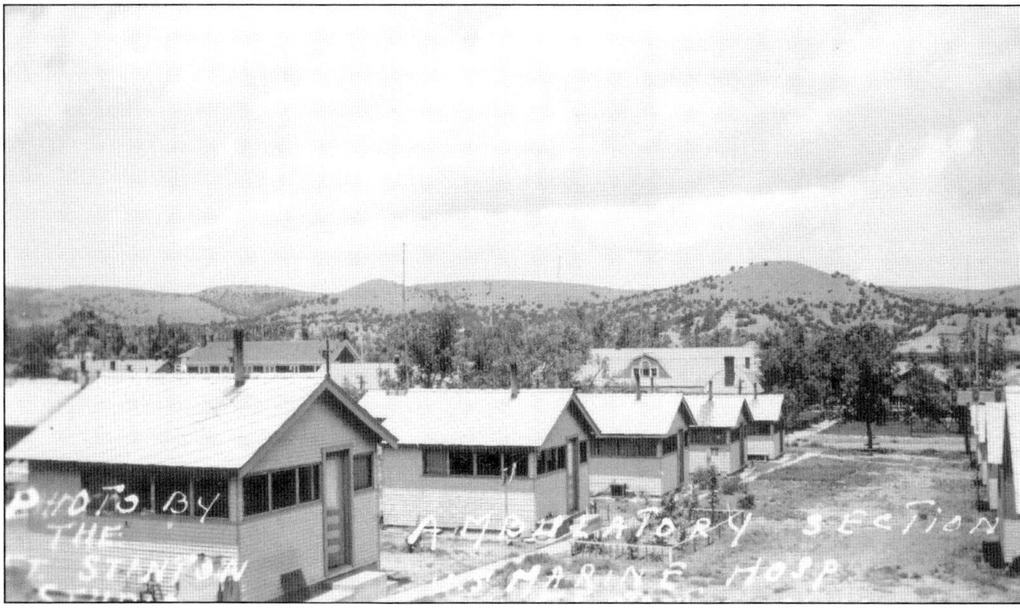

Patients whose recovery had progressed to a certain stage were allowed to live in two-man structures built east of the fort. Arranged military-style in long rows, the structures began as tent houses, but were replaced by sturdier cottages with at least a few modern conveniences. Patients often wanted to personalize their small homes, but rules even prohibited driving nails in walls. The men were eventually allowed to plant gardens. (Courtesy of Nancy Tucker.)

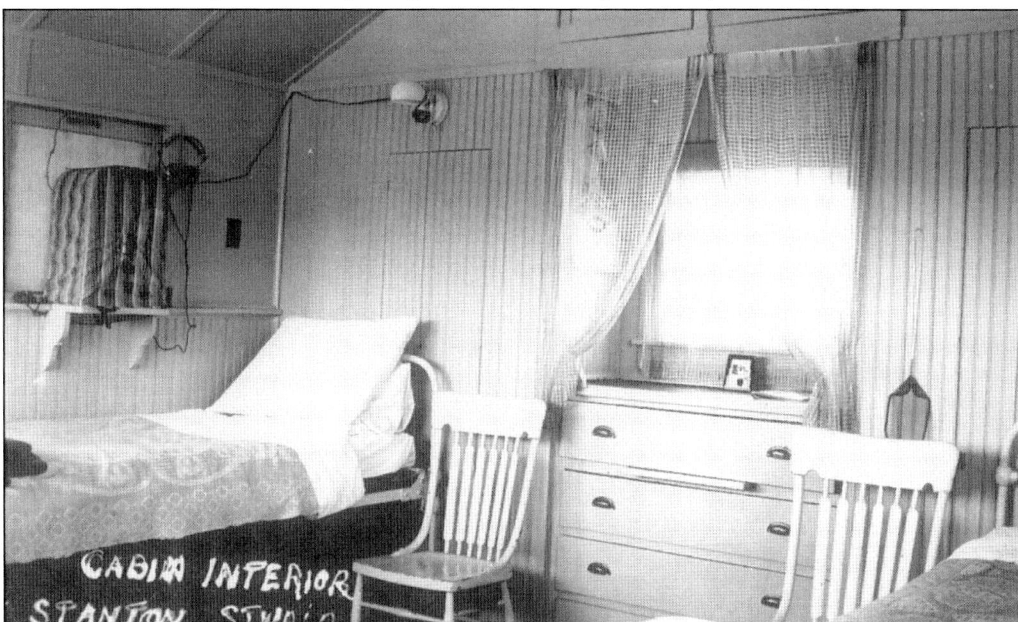

Of course, the main purpose of the cottages was to allow patients to rest with the maximum amount of clean air. Canvas window covers were only drawn down during storms and to allow them to dry if wet. Rest hours in cottages were enforced, as was lights-out at 9:00 p.m. Patients who were prescribed longer rest hours were to observe them "carefully and cheerfully," according to fort rules. (Courtesy of Donna Henderson.)

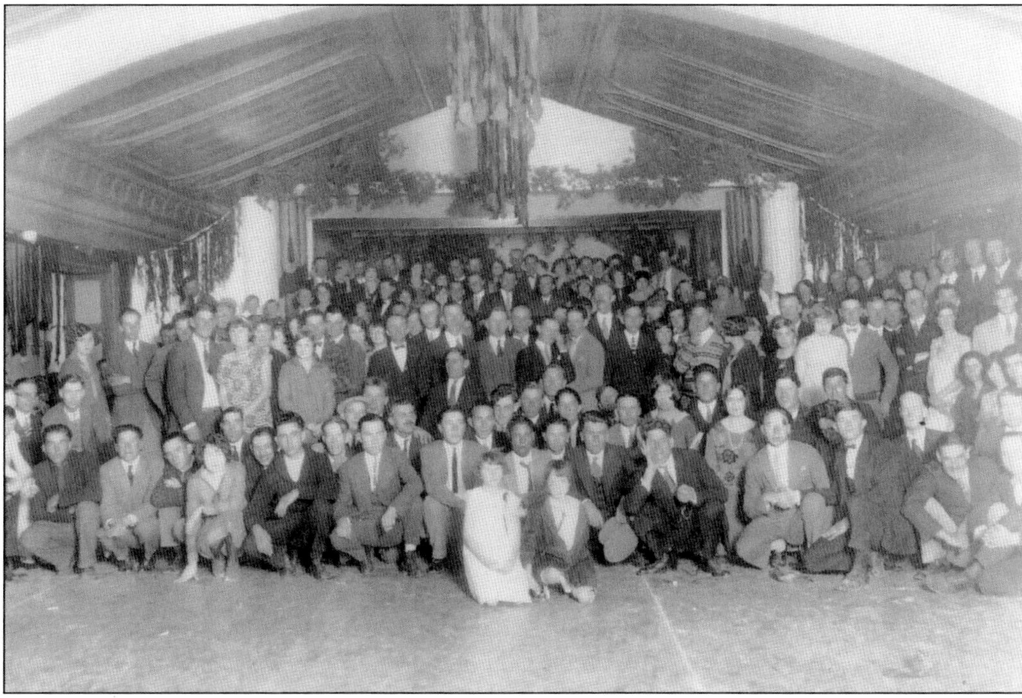

With resident doctors, nurses, staff, and their families, Fort Stanton was much like a small company town, where folks got married and raised children while otherwise employed by a single employer, the US government, for a single purpose, the care of hundreds of TB patients. By 1947, the san was described as a "complete town" with its own elementary school, Boy Scout troop, phone system, million-gallon water reservoir, and stone chapel. Its fire department responded to blazes, with the number of whistles blown indicating the designated number of the building that had caught fire. (Both, courtesy of Donna Henderson.)

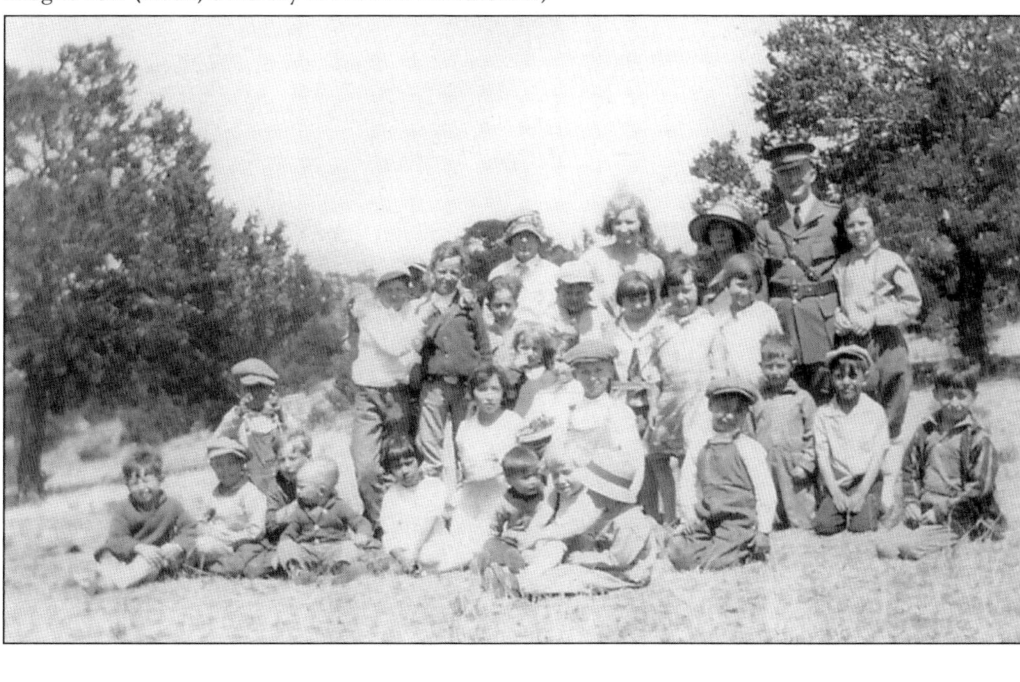

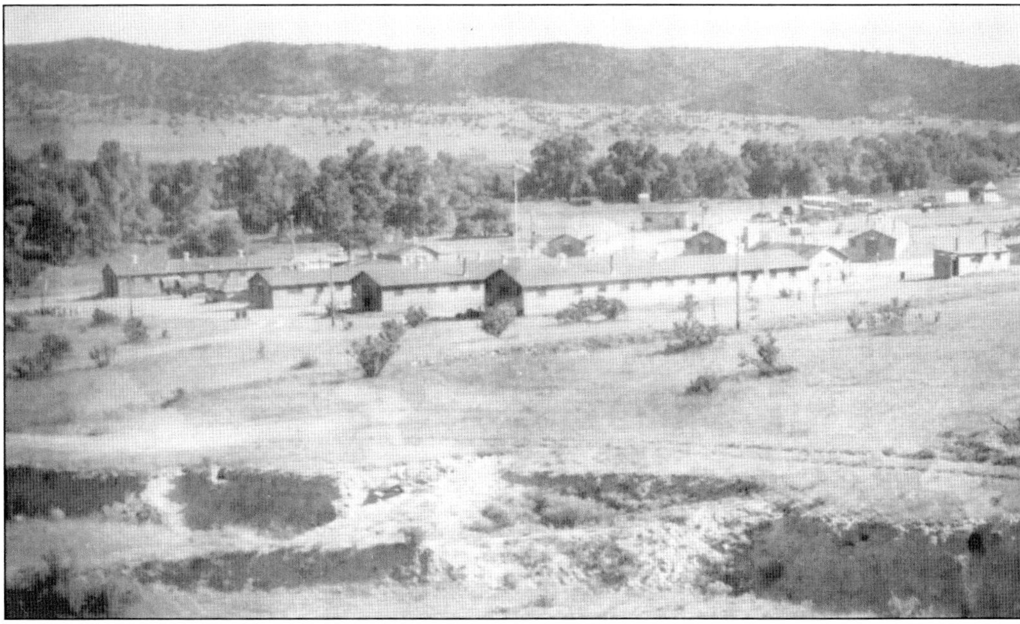

Fort Stanton benefited from two New Deal programs during the Great Depression. By 1935, a CCC camp (shown here) had been built at the foot of Round Top Hill. Some 200 young enrollees worked in the Lincoln National Forest and at the fort itself. Local men employed by the WPA built a new road from the fort to Highway 380, with a new bridge over the Rio Bonito. (Courtesy of Gary Cozzens.)

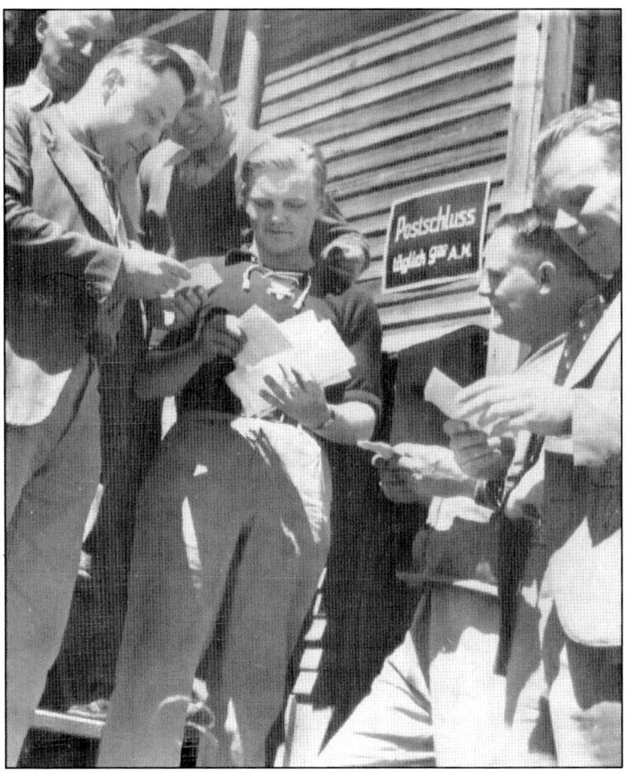

In 1939, the captain of the German liner SS *Columbus* scuttled his ship rather than surrender it at the outset of World War II. Over 400 members of the crew (including those shown here receiving mail) were detained at the site of the old CCC camp west of Fort Stanton. The Germans built a golf course, a large swimming pool, and their own farm. Japanese American internees were temporarily kept in separate quarters outside the fort.

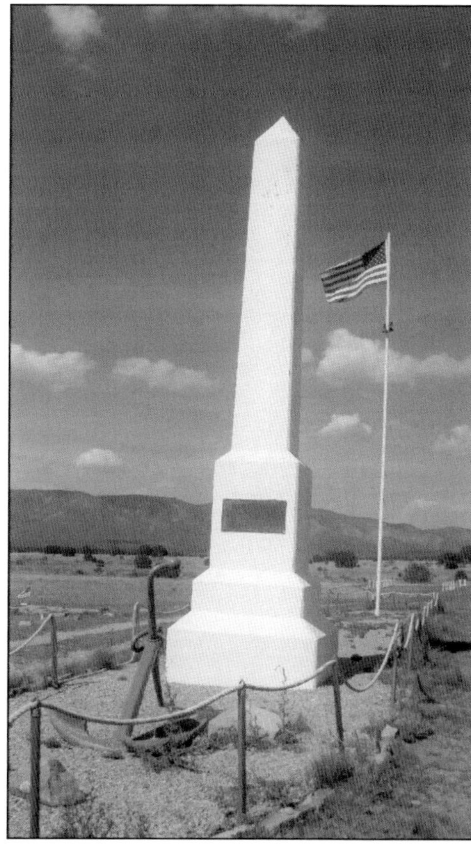

As at every san in the country, many lungers at Fort Stanton recovered their health and went on to lead happy, productive lives. Some, like Dan Kusianovich, remained at Fort Stanton to become valuable members of the staff. However, starting with John Dower in December 1899, many died at the fort, having lost their battles with TB. While many bodies were returned home for burial, Dower and 1,500 other men and women were buried at a large merchant marine cemetery a few miles east of the fort. Chaplains like Fr. James A. O'Hara, who served from 1940 to 1953, officiated at most burials.

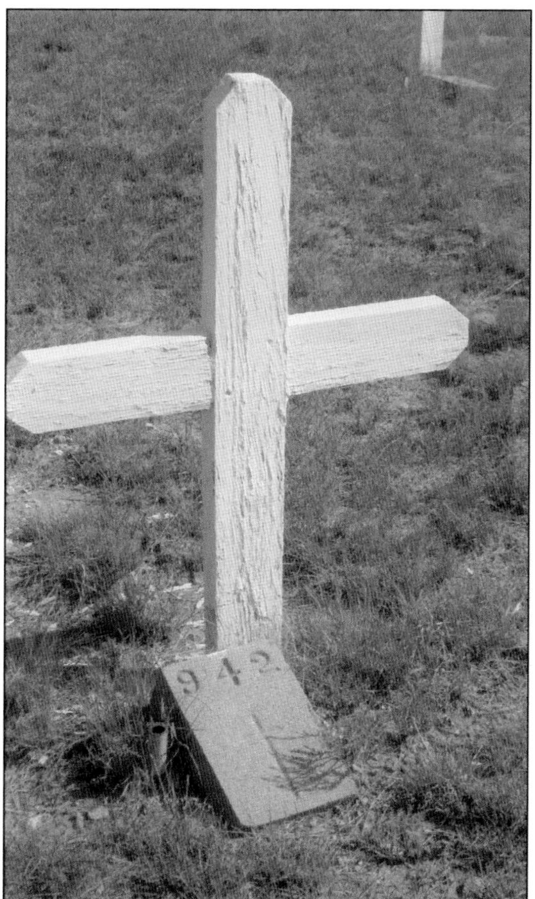

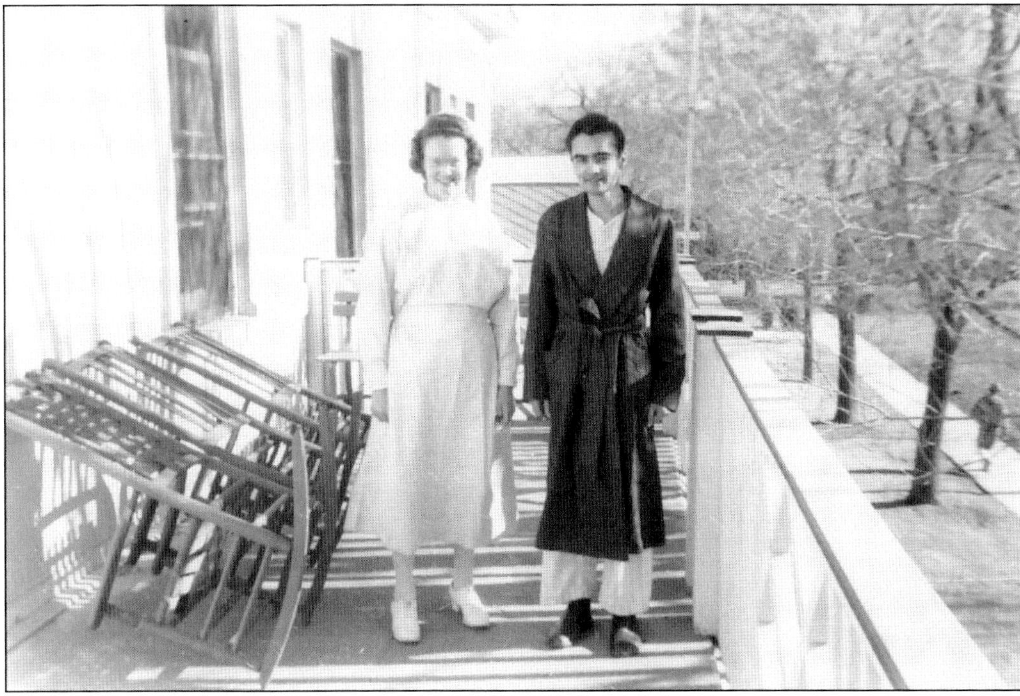

In 1947, an observer found that Fort Stanton's "friendly" population and "neatness and cleanliness" left a favorable impression even on those who were usually "the most critical of government hospitals." Unfortunately, conditions began to change when the federal government closed the merchant marines' san and turned the property over to the State of New Mexico by mid-1953. In 1964, two employees caused a scandal when they complained of excessive gambling, drinking, patient neglect, and unsafe working conditions. Other employees refuted the whistleblowers' charges, but Fort Stanton was closed within two years. Its last 90 patients were transferred to Fort Bayard. (Above, courtesy of Donna Henderson; below, courtesy of Jim Coad.)

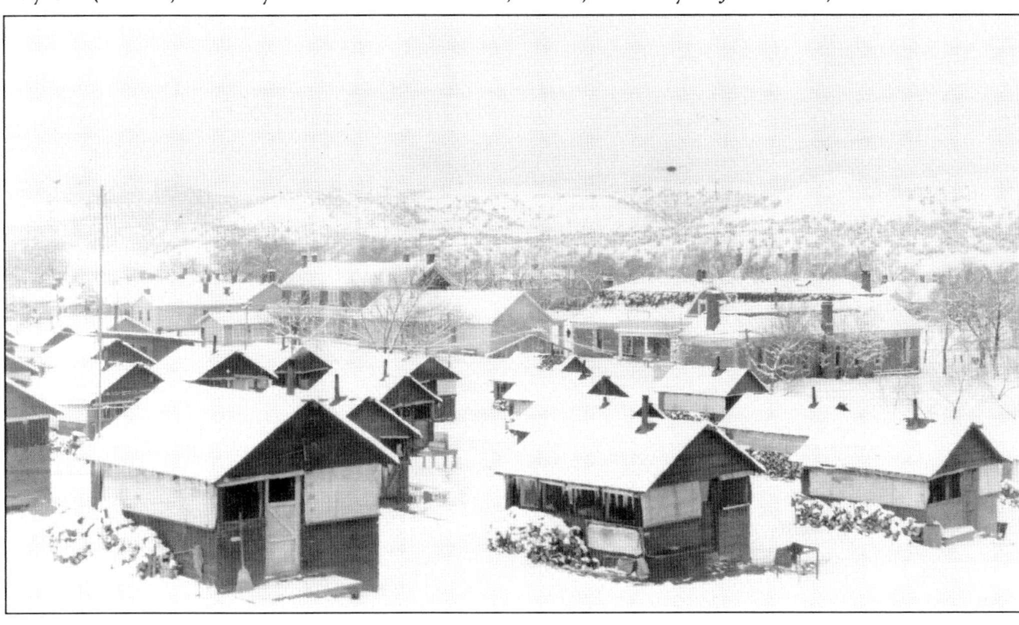

Seven

Northern New Mexico Sanatoriums

Sanatoriums in Northern New Mexico appealed to the health-seeker market with claims of an ideal climate: lots of sunshine, but none of the extreme high temperatures and powerful sandstorms of the southern half of the state. A dozen northern towns boasted at least one san. All northern sans outside of Santa Fe were privately operated, usually by a single physician, with only two sans, St. Anthony's in Las Vegas and St. Mary's in Gallup, run by religious organizations. With the exception of moderately sized St. Anthony's and Valmora, all northern sans were small, with less than 25 beds each. Located in the Sandia Mountains, three northern sans were created as lunger "resorts." Perhaps the most unusual san in state history was housed in the old Dorsey Mansion. In contrast, Valmora could claim to be the most successful, longest-existing san in the region.

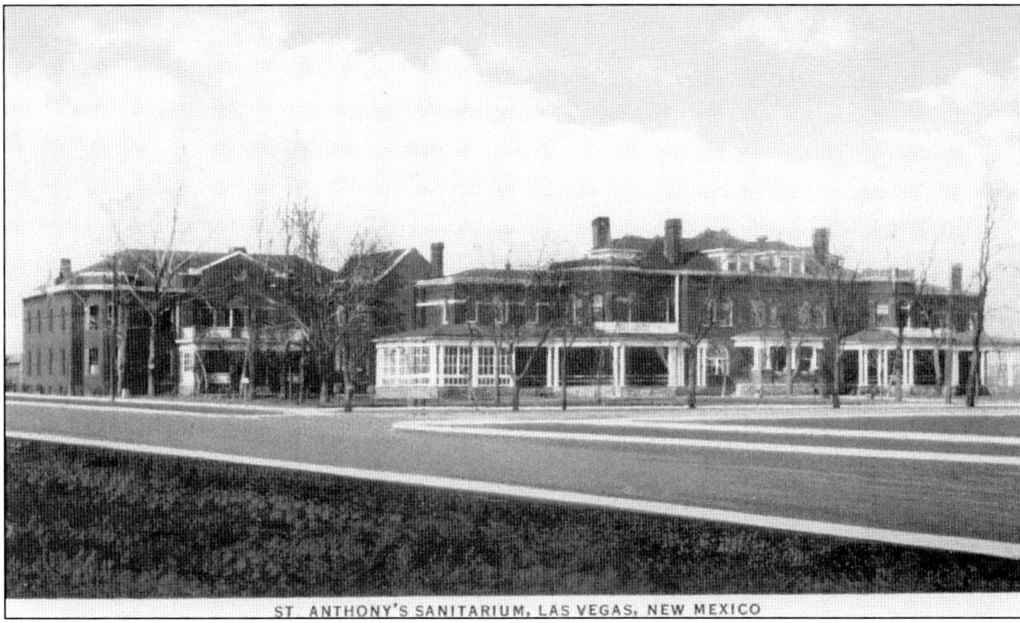
ST. ANTHONY'S SANITARIUM, LAS VEGAS, NEW MEXICO

St. Anthony's Sanatorium was dedicated in Las Vegas on January 26, 1897. The *Las Vegas Daily Optic* reported that the three-story building was the "pride of the city and the future Mecca of the invalid and healthseeker." Promotional postcards describe St. Anthony's as a "modern, fully equipped sanitarium . . . beautifully situated just within the limits of the city—in full view of the Rockies. The climate is ideal for the successful treatment of tuberculosis—dry with plenty of sunshine. The lack of humidity combined with the altitude makes it most pleasant in summer and comfortable in winter. The sanitarium is conducted by the Sisters of Charity of Leavenworth." St. Anthony's was so successful that an annex was added in 1911. With a new surgical floor built by 1918, it became a general hospital for the Las Vegas community. (Below, courtesy of Jim Coad.)

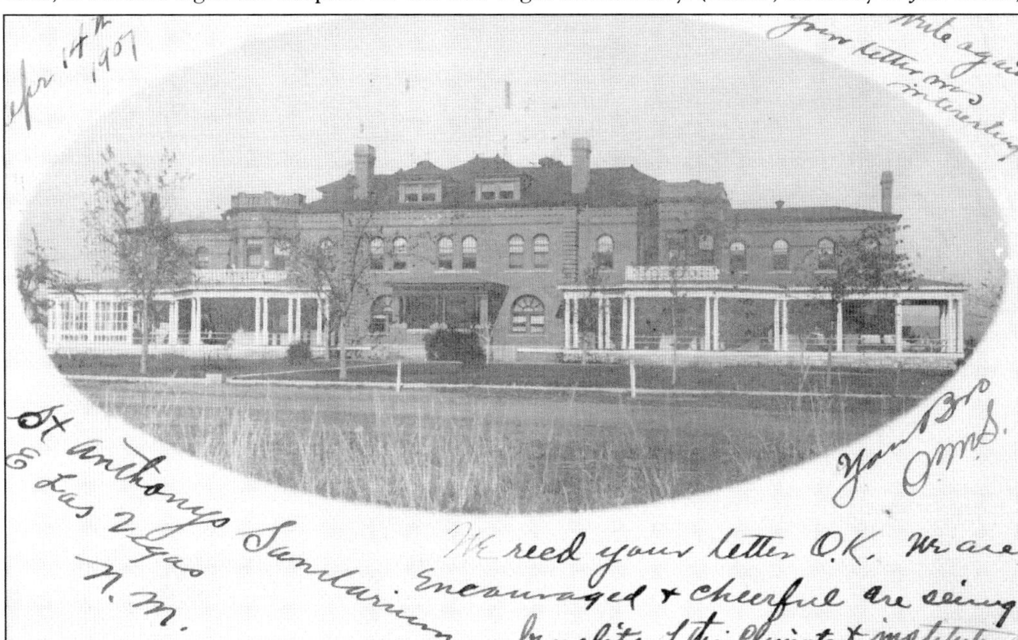
Apr 14th 1907
St Anthonys Sanitarium
E Las Vegas N.M.
Your Bro
Recd your letter O.K. We are
Encouraged + cheerful are seeing
benefits of this Climate +

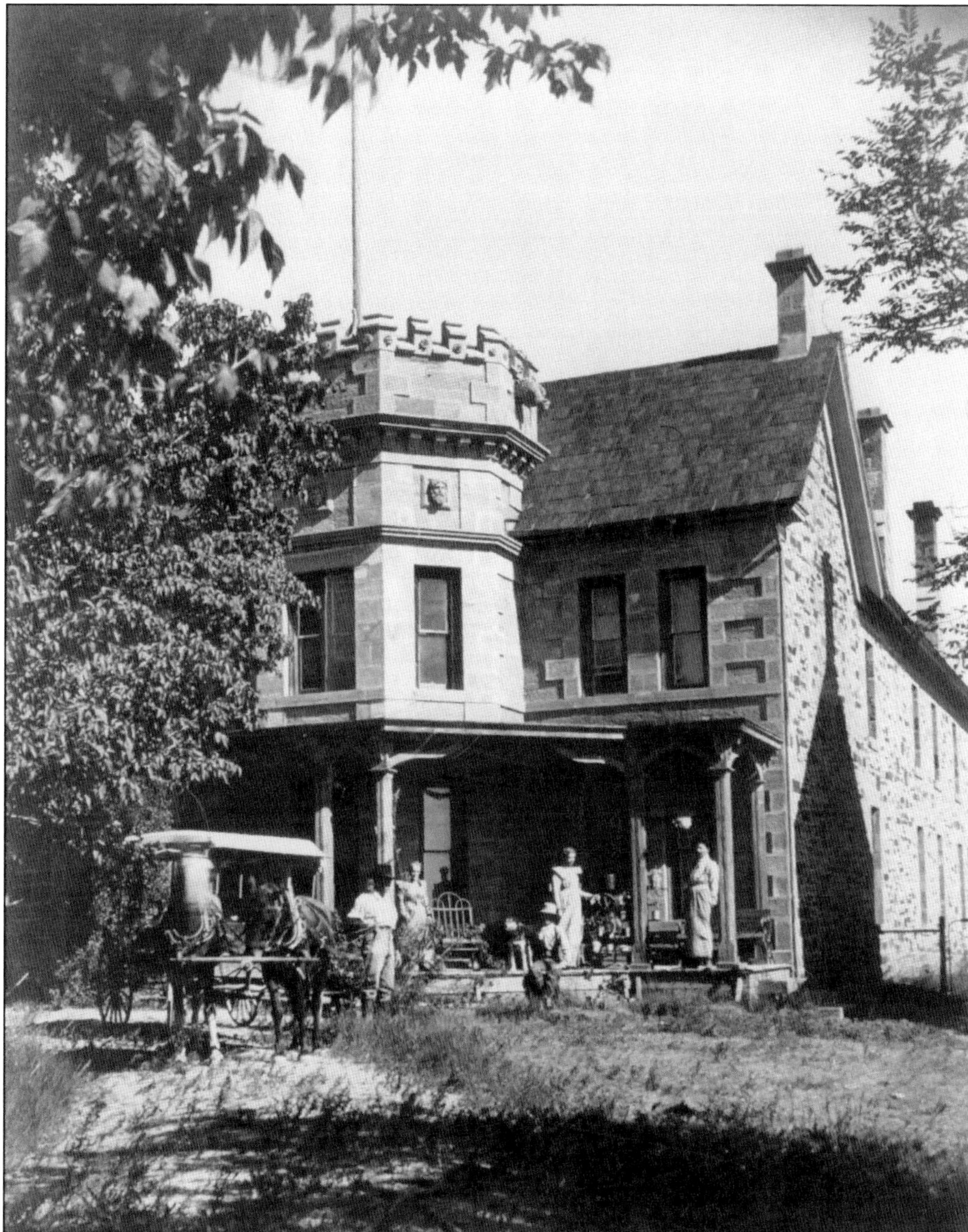

Built from 1878 to 1886, this Gothic Victorian mansion included 36 rooms, of which 9 were bedrooms. The building was owned by former Arkansas senator Stephen W. Dorsey, infamous for his involvement in the Star Route mail contract scandal. Nearly destitute by 1892, Dorsey converted his former home into a TB san. The facility operated until 1901, when he sold the entire property. It was undoubtedly the smallest, most remote, but most elaborate san in New Mexico. (Courtesy of the Museum of New Mexico, no. 43820.)

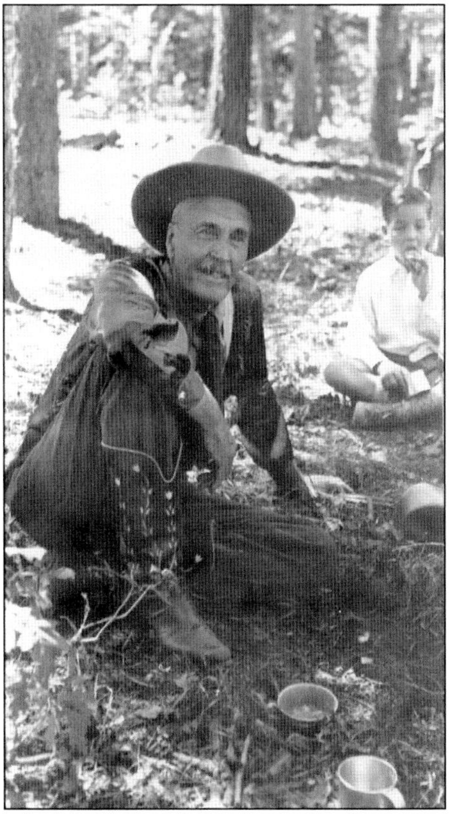

The Valmora Ranch opened in 1904. It became the Valmora Industrial Sanatorium, owned by William Townsend Brown (shown here), an English doctor who had searched the West for an ideal location to establish such an institution. In 1910, the *Las Vegas Daily Optic* reported that the sanatorium, located northeast of Las Vegas, was created for patients who could not afford more expensive sans. The institution served afflicted employees of 35 Midwest corporations. (Courtesy of Dorothy A. Simpson.)

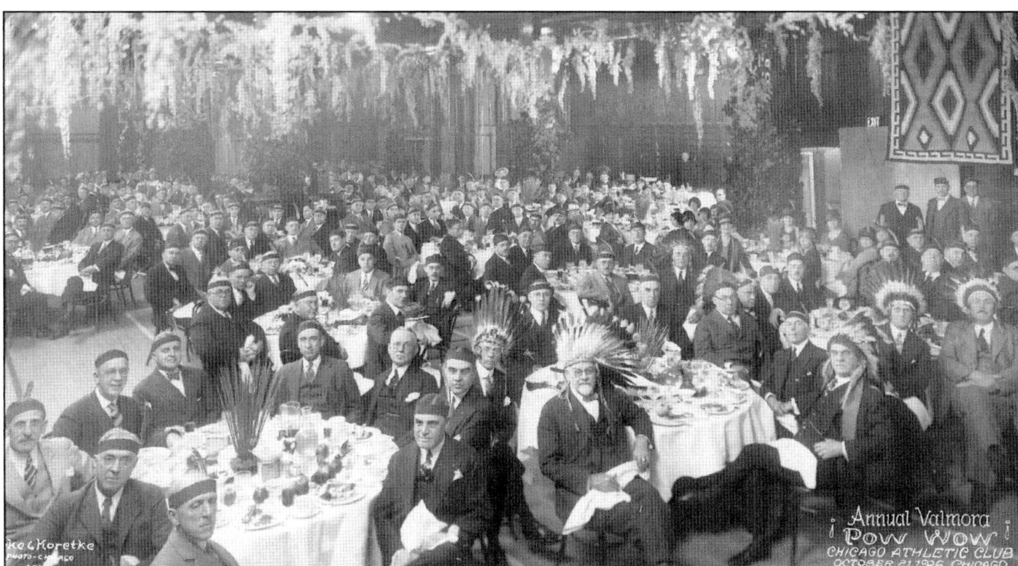
Annual Valmora
Pow Wow
CHICAGO ATHLETIC CLUB
OCTOBER 21, 1926 CHICAGO

Dr. Brown proved to be not only an excellent physician, but also an effective fundraiser back east. Gala dinners were held at large hotels, with cowboy neckerchiefs or Indian headbands for all in attendance. With dependable financial support, the san grew to include 29 cottages, a recreation hall, a post office, vegetable gardens, a ranch, and a dairy. (Courtesy of Special Collections, University of New Mexico's Health Science Library.)

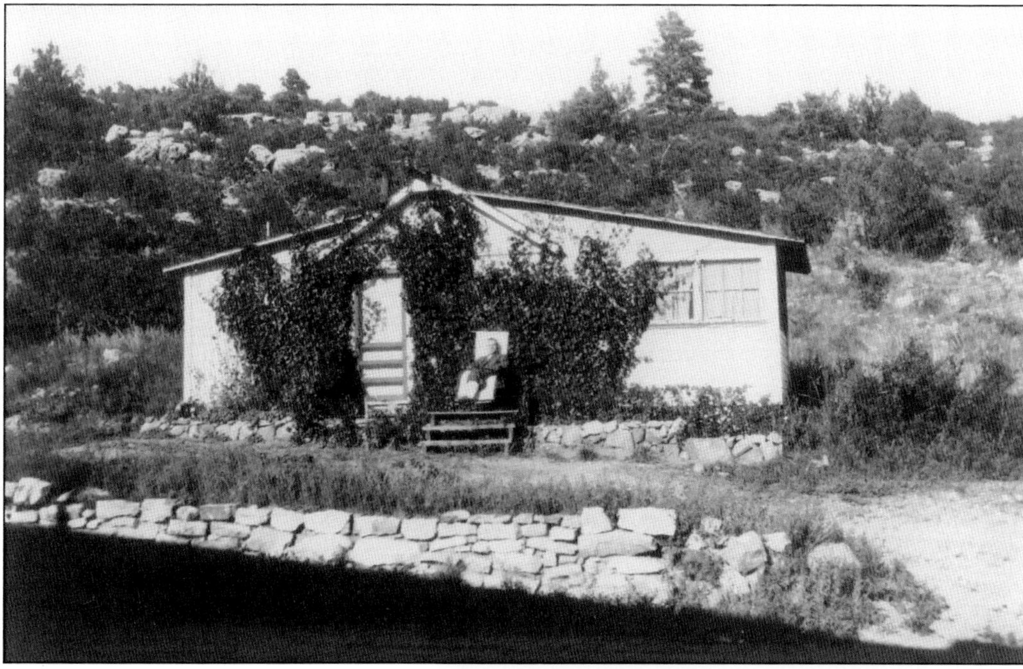

Dr. Brown required that each new patient "cheerfully" sign off that he or she promised to live by Brown's 14 rules, including no drinking or smoking, no leaving the san without permission, no profane language, no gambling, no spitting (except in provided pocket cuspidors), and no talking about one's symptoms. Rule No. 8 banned "private associations" of male and female patients. (Courtesy of Special Collections, UNM Health Sciences Library.)

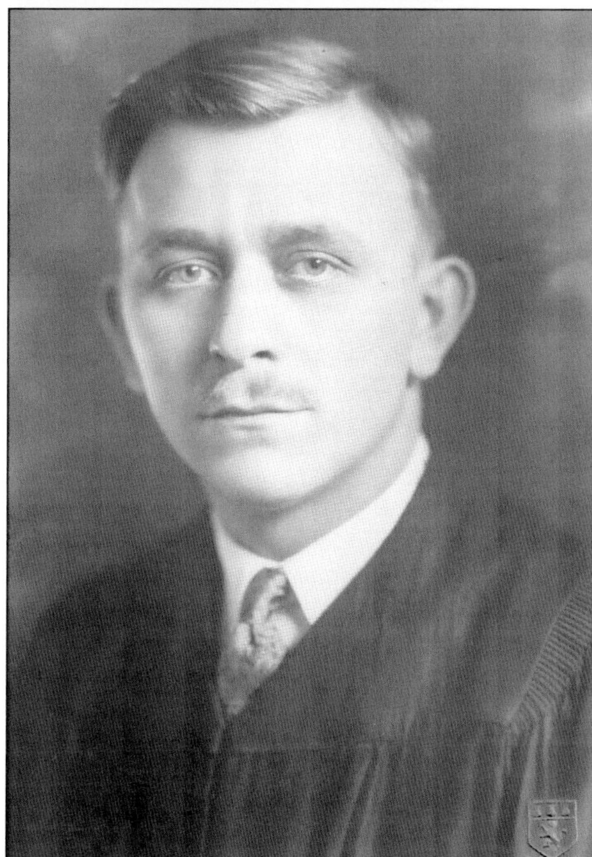

The san continued to grow with the arrival of Carl Gellenthien (shown here), who had contracted TB while studying medicine. After convalescing at Valmora, Gellenthien finished his medical degree in 1926. With fond memories of Valmora and a certain young dietitian (Dr. Brown's daughter, Alice), Gellenthien returned, becoming the san's medical director. "Dr. G" married Alice and assumed full responsibility for the san when Brown died in 1935. (Courtesy of Dorothy A. Simpson.)

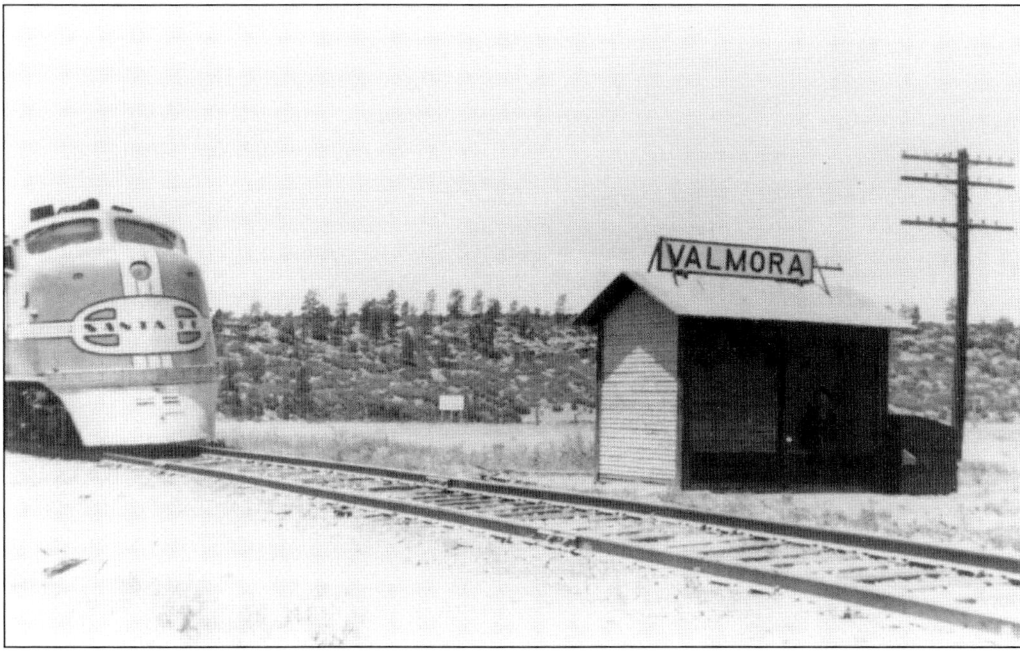

Patients came to Valmora from nearly every state in the union, plus 15 European and South American countries. Dr. G kept a world map, covered with red dots, each representing a hometown of one or more of his patients. According to historian Dorothy A. Simpson, over 5,000 patients were treated at Valmora from 1905 to 1931. The longest stay was seven years; the average stay was two. Valmora claimed to have the lowest death rate and the highest percentage of cures of all registered sans in the United States. (Both, courtesy of Special Collections, UNM Health Sciences Library.)

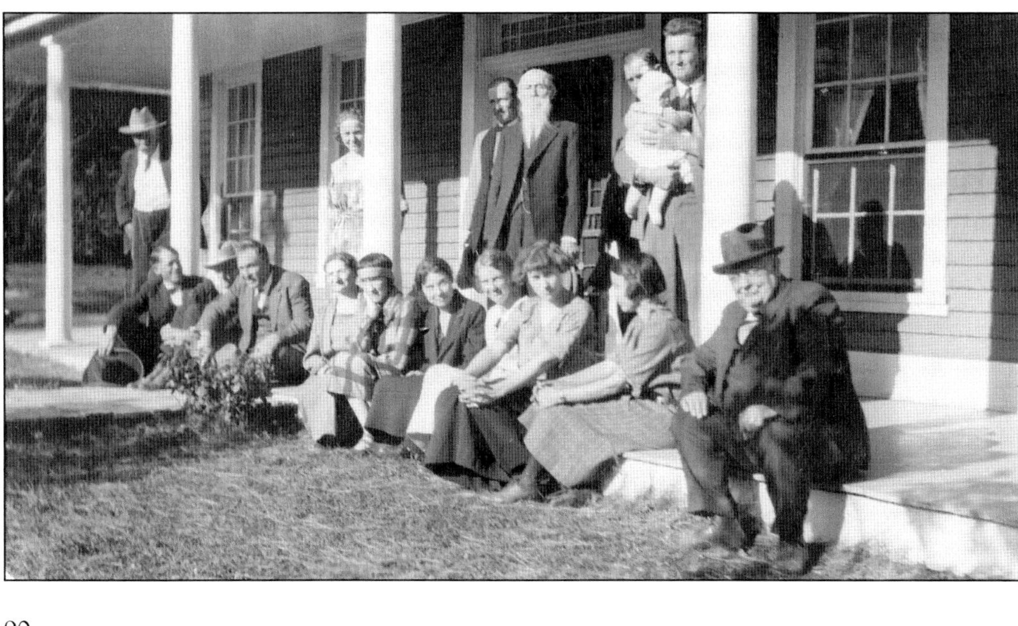

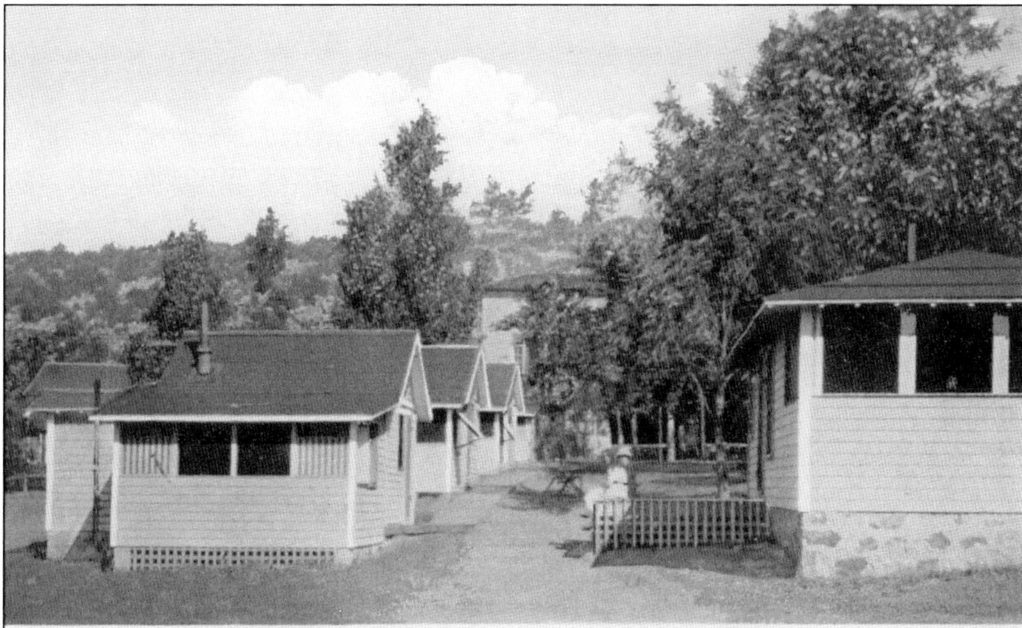
COTTAGES, VALMORA SANATORIUM, VALMORA, NEW MEXICO. 107573

Valmora's private cottages allowed for maximum air ventilation and comfort. Pleased with his cottage life, the "Bedridden Bard" wrote the poem "Us TBs," included in Dorothy A. Simpson's *Valmora: A Place of Inspiration:* "We are forced to live in a beautiful state / In order the bugs to eradicate. / The people are fine and the food is good/ We're just a happy neighborhood. / The nurses are nice and try to please / The slightest whims of us TBs . . . / We can read or write or snooze away / There's lots to do to pass the day. / Bridge or chess or other games / Or conversations with pretty dames. / We get all this at very low fees / So life is kind to us TBs."

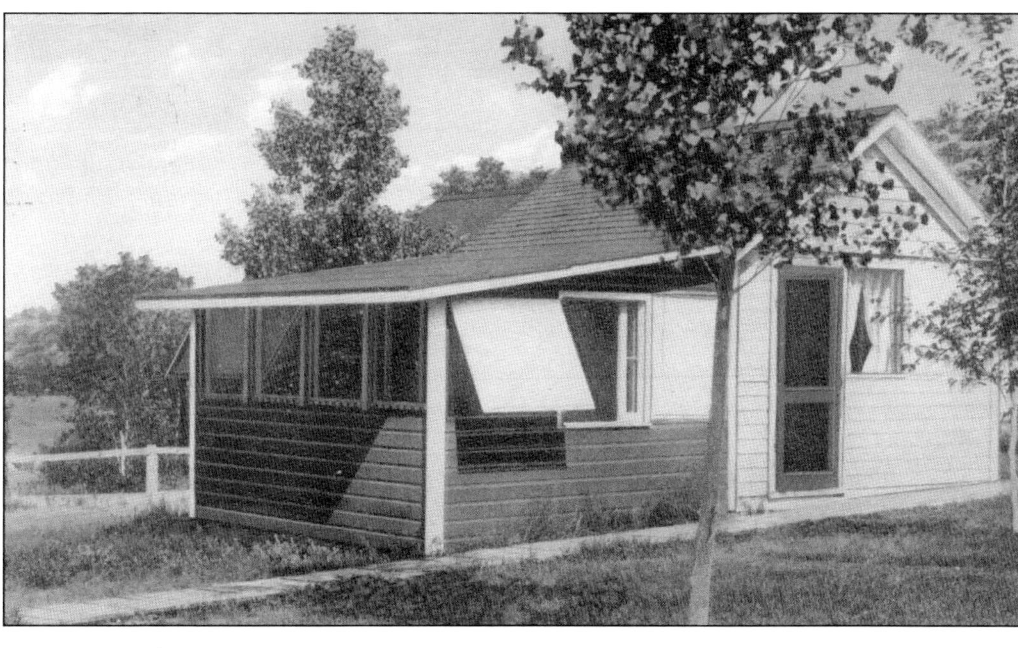

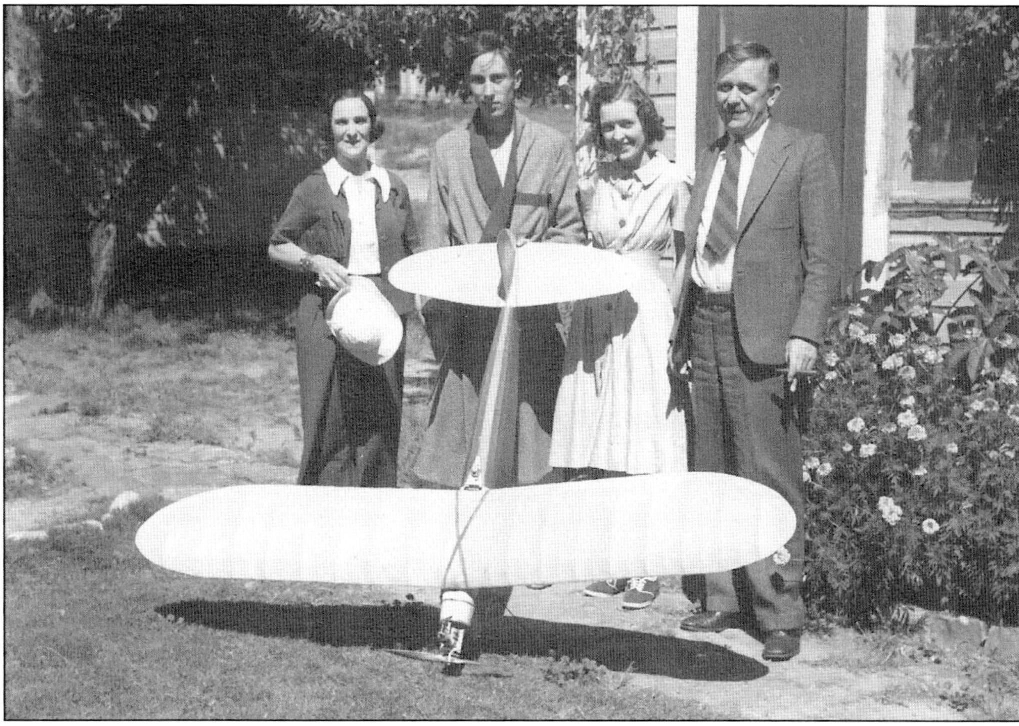

Dr. Brown and Dr. G (far right) stressed the importance of occupational therapy and creative activities as essential parts of their patients' recovery. Patients were taught everything from music and art to pottery and moccasin making. Some continued their careers while at Valmora. The popular Vivian "Johnnie" Johnson (second from right) served as the san's secretary. Recovered patients included successful photographers, musicians, artists, businessmen, and at least one trading-post operator. (Courtesy of Dorothy A. Simpson.)

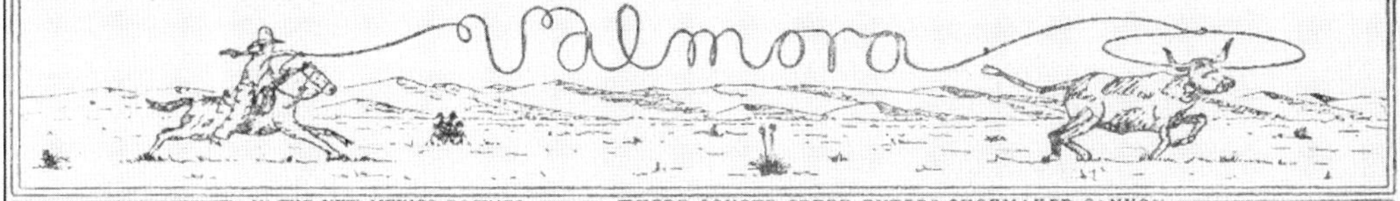
Valmora
IN THE NEW MEXICO ROCKIES
WHERE COYOTE CREEK ENTERS SHOEMAKER CANYON

Many writers honed their skills by working on the san's six newspapers, filling them with local news, jokes, and original fiction. Starting in 1925 with the *Val Moran*, succeeding newspapers included the *Valmora Tattler* and the *Valmora Chatter*. While a patient at the san, William Guinn started to write his Western novel *Death Lies Deep*, using Dr. G as the inspiration for the fictional Doc Freeman. (Courtesy of Special Collections, UNM Health Sciences Library.)

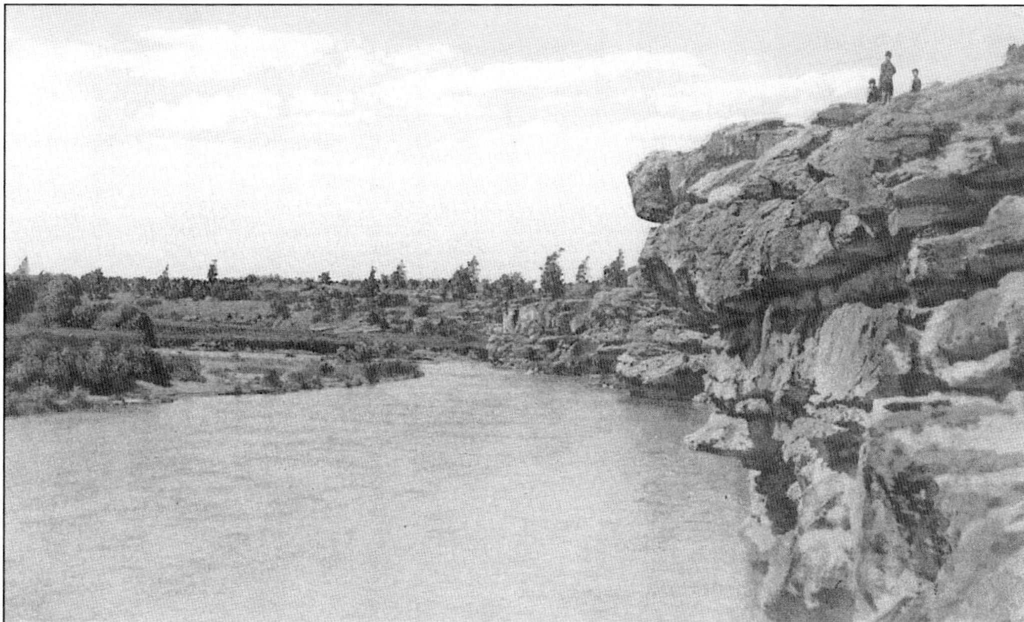

MORA RIVER, NEAR VALMORA SANATORIUM, VALMORA, NEW MEXICO 107575

Located in a beautiful valley, Valmora offered opportunities that made patients feel they were on vacation from their daily routines. Within walking distance of the san, patients discovered arrowheads, shards of Indian pottery, and ancient petroglyphs in nearby caves. Other patients traveled in the san's "chariot" to shop or, in one case, attend a wedding in Santa Fe. Las Vegas merchants held an annual "Valmora Day," with discounts for all lungers.

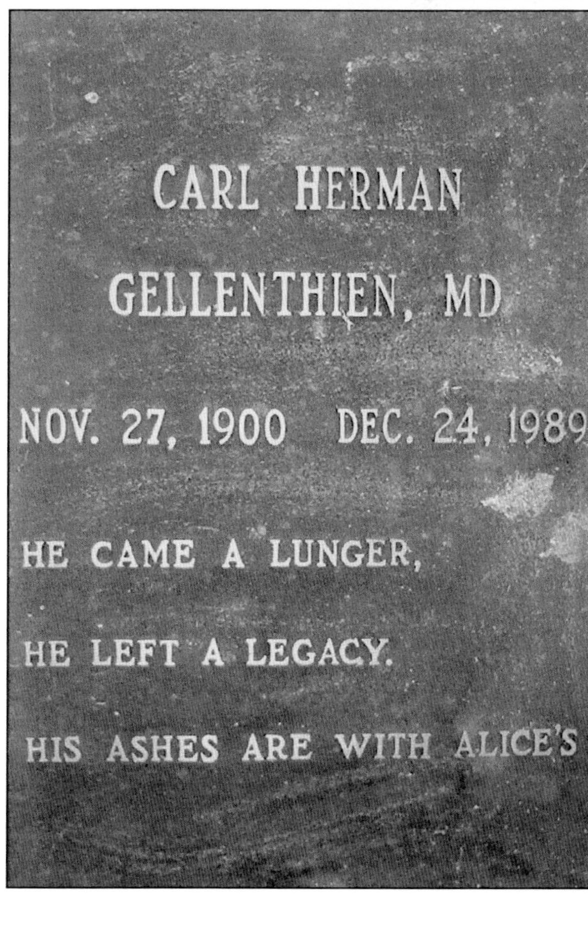

About a dozen patients still lived at the popular san as late as 1954. Dr. G remained in practice long after the san closed, serving the residents of the surrounding rural communities until his death at the age of 89 in 1989. As he often said, "It's been a great life." A three-day auction in 1991 disposed of everything at the san, from wicker wheelchairs to feet warmers.

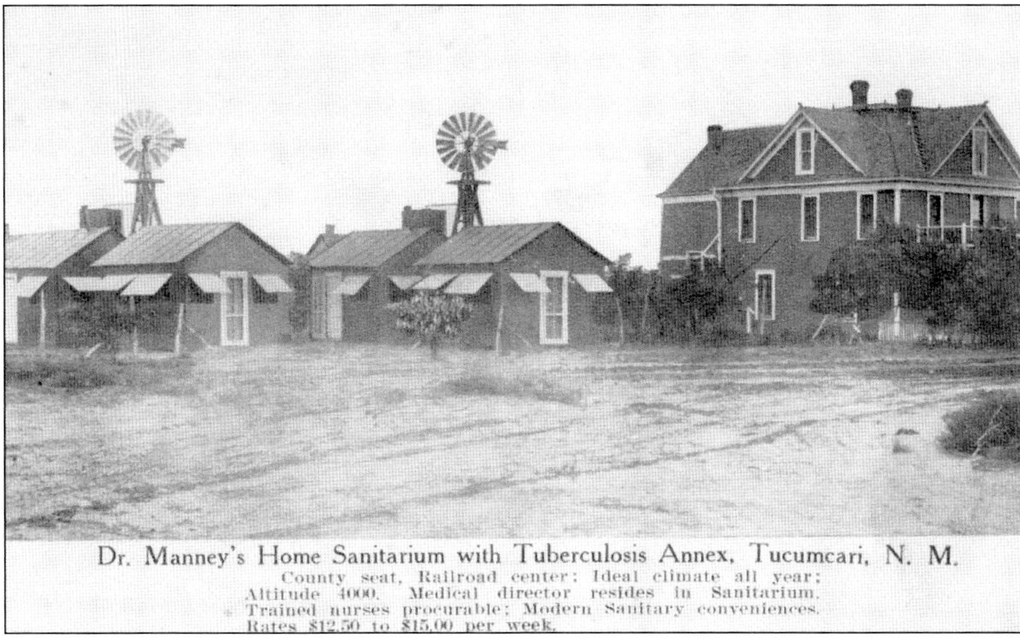
Dr. Manney's Home Sanitarium with Tuberculosis Annex, Tucumcari, N. M.
County seat, Railroad center: Ideal climate all year:
Altitude 4000. Medical director resides in Sanitarium.
Trained nurses procurable: Modern Sanitary conveniences.
Rates $12.50 to $15.00 per week.

Tucumcari's Dr. John E. Manney opened his 16-room home sanitarium in 1907. The son of an ex–Confederate soldier who later joined the Ku Klux Klan, Dr. Manney probably ran a segregated san. In response to such segregation, John Cott opened an African American sanatorium east of Silver City, reportedly the first of its kind nationally. Albuquerque's Booker T. Washington Memorial Sanatorium opened by 1920. Unfortunately, neither institution lasted very long. (Courtesy of Nancy Tucker.)

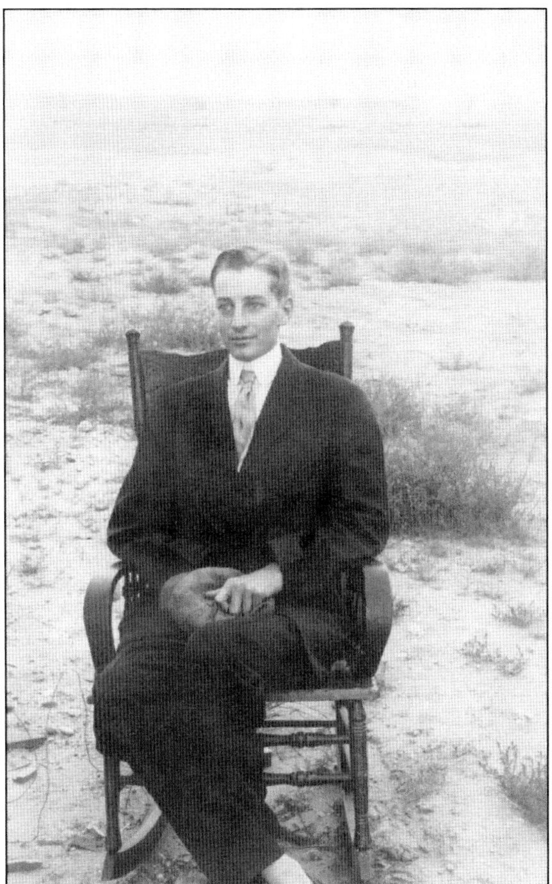

Lunger Larry Glasebrook arrived in New Mexico in 1912 with a diagnosis that he had no more than four months to live. Despite this prediction, in 1914, he and four fellow health-seekers established a small lungers' resort in the Sandia Mountains, with two large tents and an appropriate name, Kamp Killgloom. The "kamp" remained open for summer guests until a permanent site made year-round occupancy possible by 1920. (Courtesy of Penny Hobbie.)

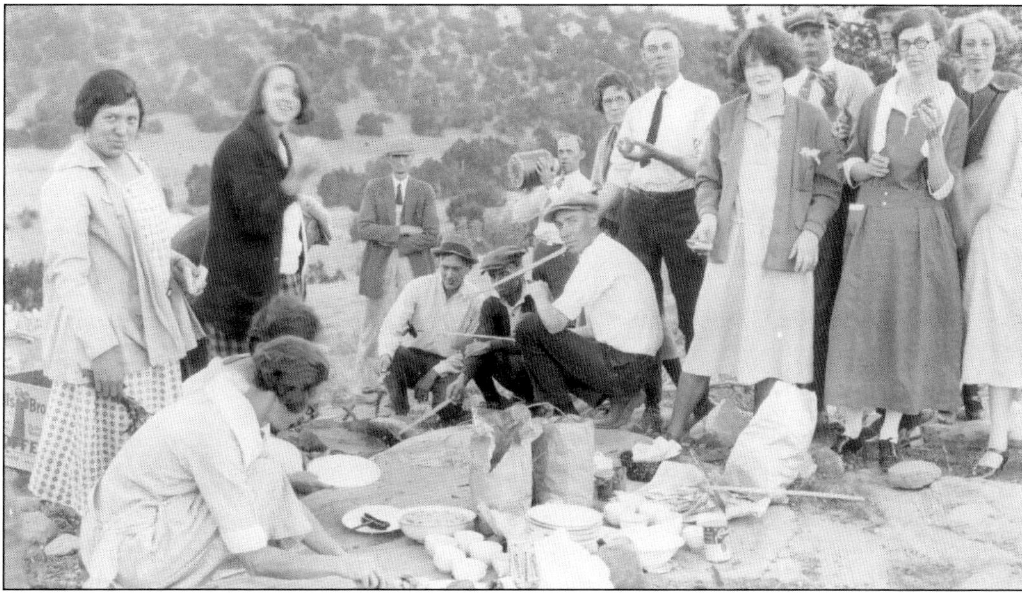

These photographs of guests at the Well Country Camp suggest that any of them could have written a *Health City Sun* article titled "Learn to Let Troubles Go." Guests enjoyed frequent picnics, so-called tacky parties, and similarly amusing events. Larry Glasebrook also published the *Killgloom Gazette* (later known as the *Herald of the Well Country*), whose wit and humor became so popular among fellow lungers that its monthly circulation reached 1,000 copies. Glasebrook claimed to be uniquely qualified to publish the *Gazette*, because he had many degrees (over 98.6), belonged to the Eta Raw Egg fraternity, and sang in the One Lung Glee Club. According to historian Mike Smith, a local resident once said, "If I had stumbled into [Kamp Killgloom], I would have thought it was a mental home, not a TB place." (Both, courtesy of Penny Hobbie.)

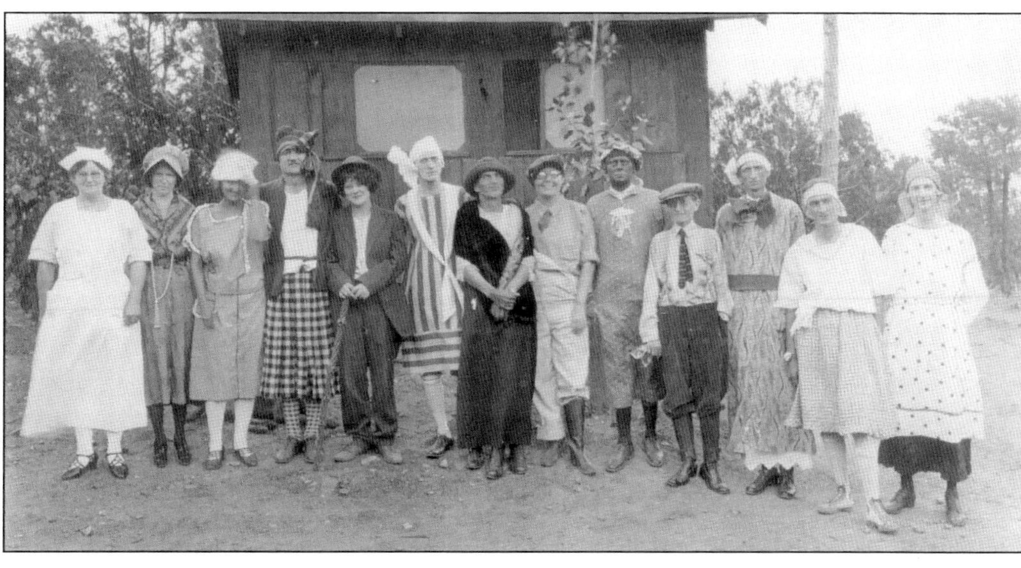

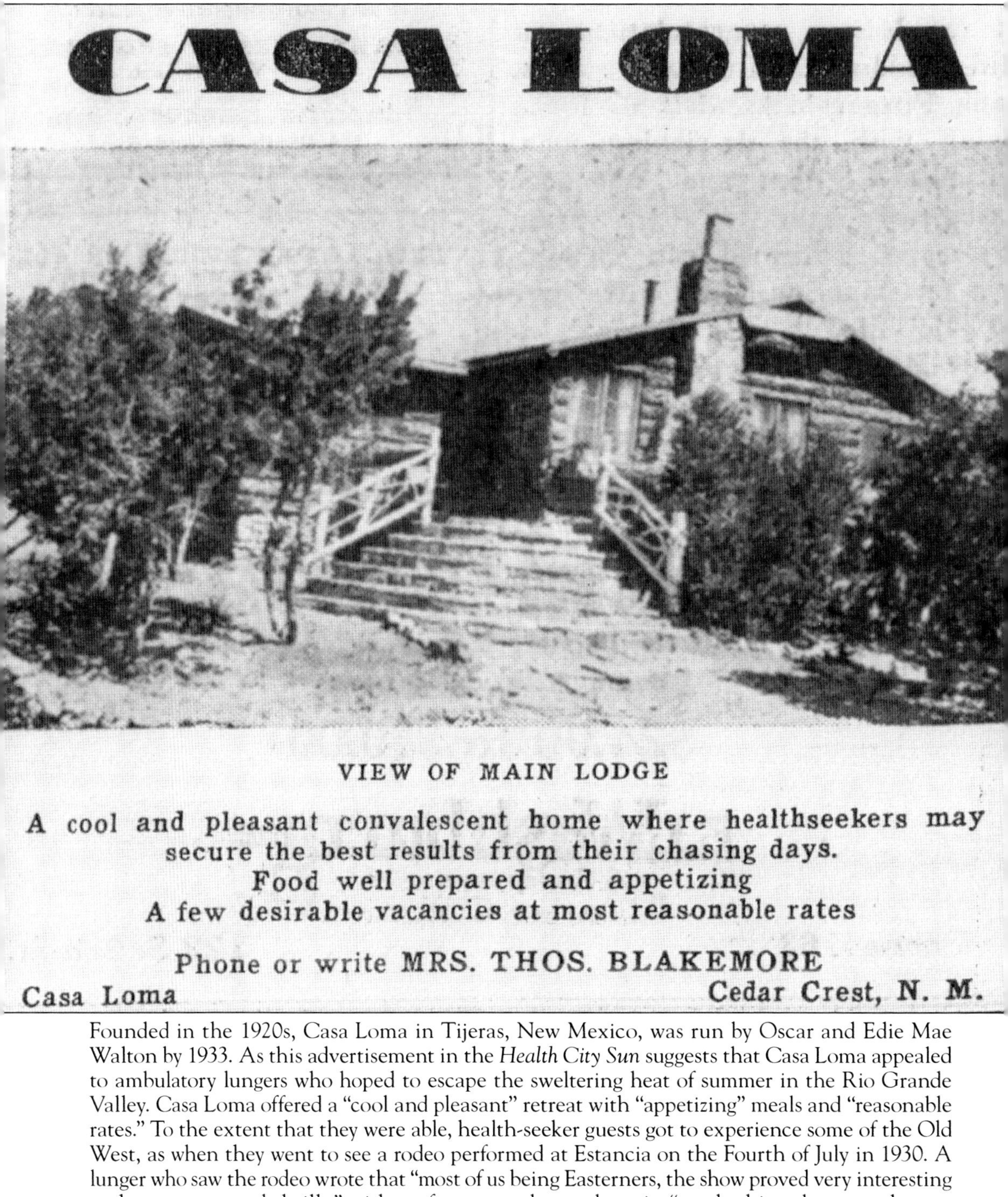

Founded in the 1920s, Casa Loma in Tijeras, New Mexico, was run by Oscar and Edie Mae Walton by 1933. As this advertisement in the *Health City Sun* suggests that Casa Loma appealed to ambulatory lungers who hoped to escape the sweltering heat of summer in the Rio Grande Valley. Casa Loma offered a "cool and pleasant" retreat with "appetizing" meals and "reasonable rates." To the extent that they were able, health-seeker guests got to experience some of the Old West, as when they went to see a rodeo performed at Estancia on the Fourth of July in 1930. A lunger who saw the rodeo wrote that "most of us being Easterners, the show proved very interesting and gave us several thrills," with performances by cowboys in "gaudy shirts, large sombreros, chaparajos, and spurs."

Eight

SOUTHERN NEW MEXICO SANATORIUMS

Southern New Mexico seemed ideally suited to serve health-seekers in search of clean, dry air in a moderate, year-round climate; brochures documented the average number of days of sunshine (362) and average daytime temperature (76 degrees) in the region. Sunkist and Sunnyside sanatoriums marketed their greatest asset in their chosen names. In all, 10 communities catered to the health-seeker industry, with from one sanatorium to as many as six (in Silver City). Hot Springs, now Truth or Consequences, also appealed to health-seekers, emphasizing the healing powers of its spas for a wide range of ailments. Most sans were privately owned, usually by a single physician, with three sans run by nuns of the Catholic Church. The government ran three institutions—the state san north of Socorro; Fort Bayard; and Fort Stanton. Private sans varied in size, from the very smallest in Lincoln and Carlsbad, to the largest in Alamogordo and Silver City. Most sans were isolated, helping to alleviate local fears of catching the dreaded disease.

Although each town vied with all others for the distinction of providing the best opportunity for recovery from TB, Silver City far outdid its regional competition. The *Silver City Enterprise*'s masthead went so far as to include the assertion that Silver City had "The Best Climate in the World—A Paradise for Consumptives." With appeals like these, a 1913 health survey reports that more than half of Silver City residents are health-seekers or their relatives. The town's TB boom occurred just as its economy needed it the most, after the collapse of the silver industry in 1893 and before large-scale copper mining began in 1910.

Many Silver City lungers lived on their own in private residences. Future Arizona congresswoman Isabella Greenway and her first husband, lunger Robert Munro-Ferguson, lived in the Burro Mountains, where they were visited by friends, including Franklin and Eleanor Roosevelt. The town's lunger population included New Mexico's most famous health-seeker, Catherine Antrim, Billy the Kid's mother, who succumbed to TB in 1874, long before the first san opened for business in the community.

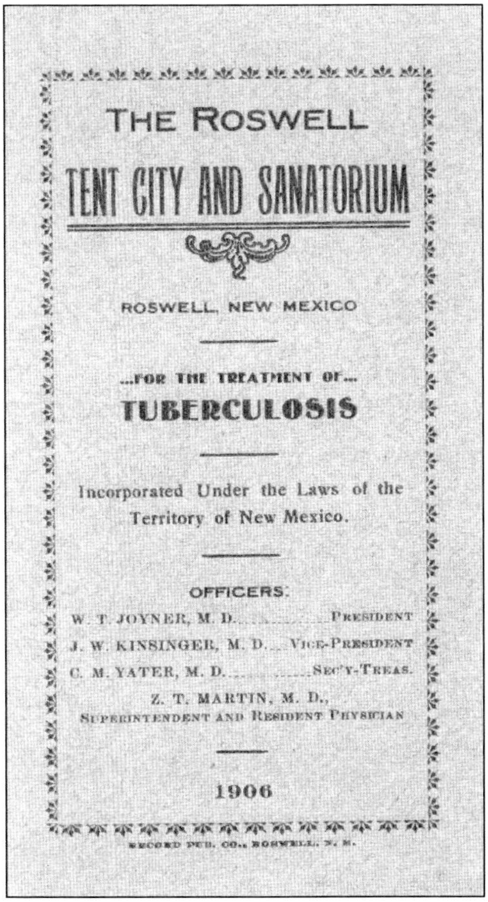

THE ROSWELL

TENT CITY AND SANATORIUM

ROSWELL, NEW MEXICO

...FOR THE TREATMENT OF...

TUBERCULOSIS

Incorporated Under the Laws of the Territory of New Mexico.

OFFICERS:

W. T. JOYNER, M. D. .... PRESIDENT

J. W. KINSINGER, M. D. .... VICE-PRESIDENT

C. M. YATER, M. D. .... SEC'Y-TREAS.

Z. T. MARTIN, M. D., SUPERINTENDENT AND RESIDENT PHYSICIAN

1906

RECORD PUB. CO., ROSWELL, N. M.

A Roswell businessman visited the Sunmount Tent City in Santa Fe and returned home convinced that a similar facility would work well in northwest Roswell. Endorsed by Roswell's Commercial Club and largely financed by Dr. C.M. Yater, the colony sanatorium opened with 20 tents in 1905. For $10 a week, patients received a "nicely furnished tent cottage, board, a supervision of diet, exercise, and advice." (Courtesy of Nancy Tucker.)

By 1904, the largely Protestant population of Roswell hoped to open a hospital and sanatorium in its growing community. Local leaders asked the Catholic Sisters of the Sorrowful Mother for assistance. The sisters agreed and, by 1905, a committee, including several nuns, visited businesses to raise $15,000 for the project. Less reputable institutions, like saloons, were asked to contribute "without the assistance of the sisters."

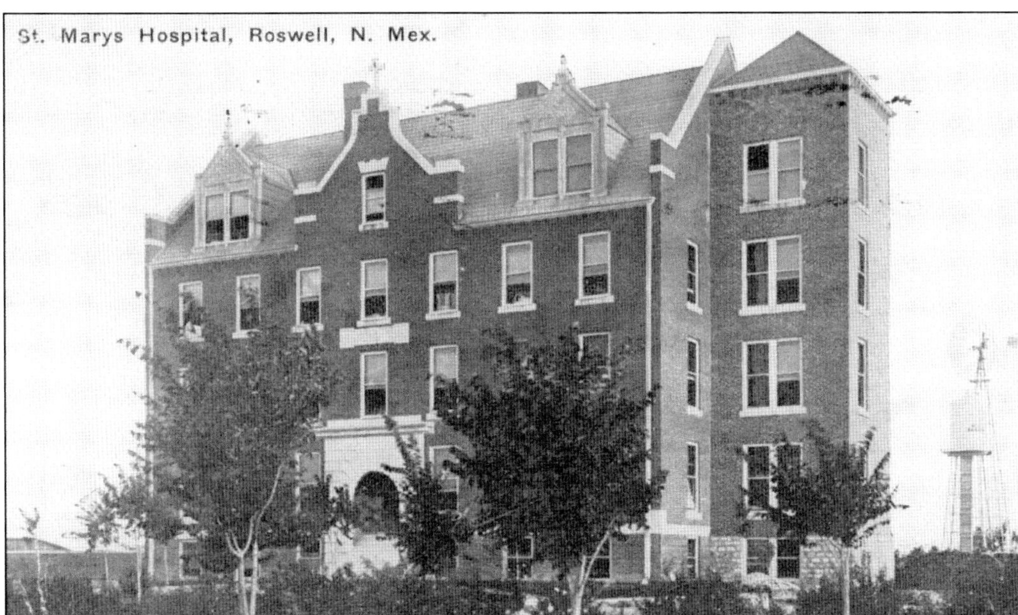

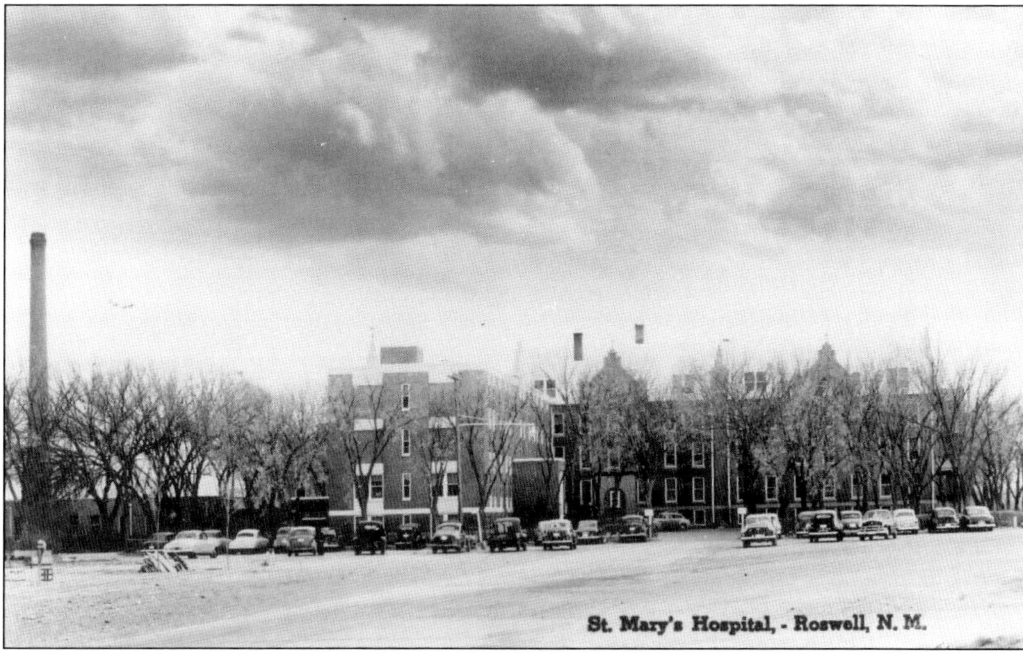

St. Mary's three-story structure (above) was built on 10 acres of ranchland south of town. The 26-bed hospital's formal opening took place on June 1, 1906. Local residents contributed money, crops, and a horse and buggy to transport the nuns to town. But fear of TB soon set in, causing people to become wary of the new institution. The hospital reacted by adding an isolated 12-room wing for bedridden lungers and 20 tents for ambulatory lungers by 1908. Lungers flocked to Roswell until the Great Depression, when St. Mary's finally closed its san. St. Mary's operated as a general hospital (below) until 1989, when it became part of the Eastern New Mexico Medical Center. (Above, courtesy of Jim Coad.)

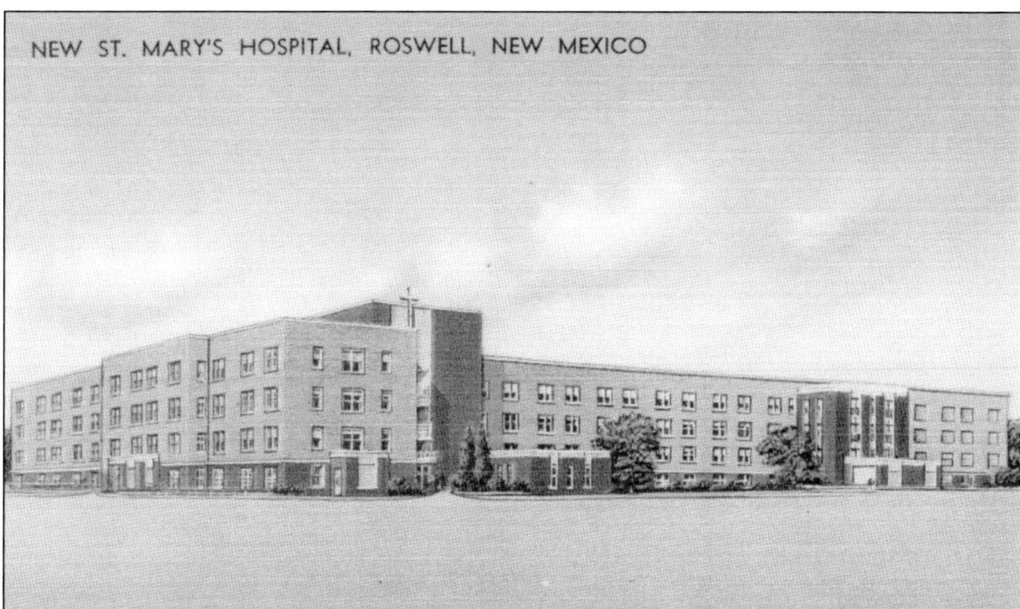

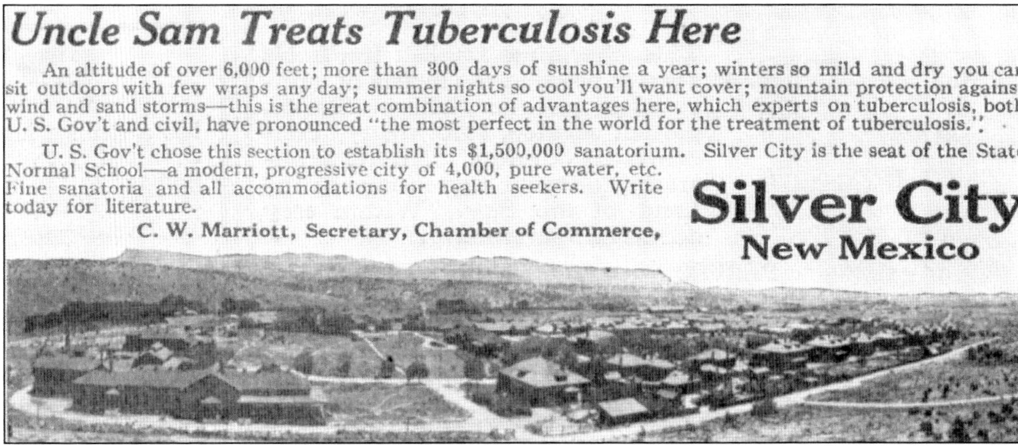

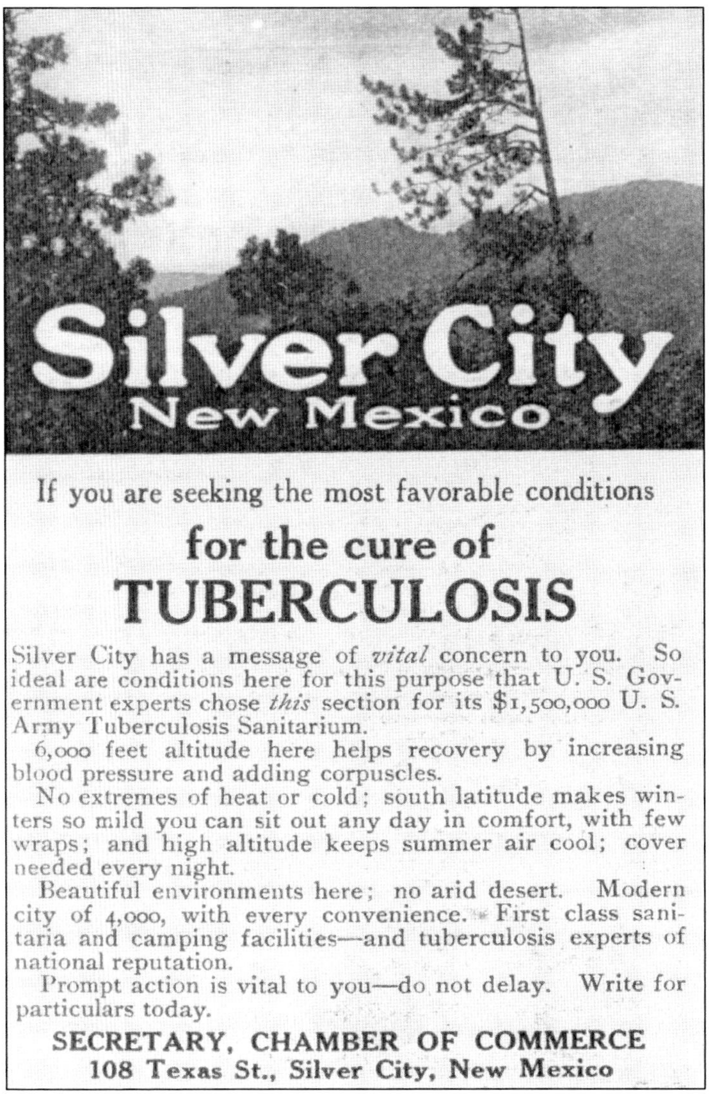

The Silver City Chamber of Commerce published advertisements in periodicals across the United States to promote the community's number one asset at the turn of the 20th century. The promotions claim that Silver City offers "ideal conditions" for the cure of tuberculosis: high altitude, plenty of sunshine, moderate temperature, TB experts, first-class sans, and beautiful surroundings. The chamber boasted that the area was so perfect that "U.S. Government experts" chose it to establish a $1.5 million Army sanatorium. As with any good salesman, the chamber told health-seekers that "prompt action is vital to you—do not delay. Write for particulars today."

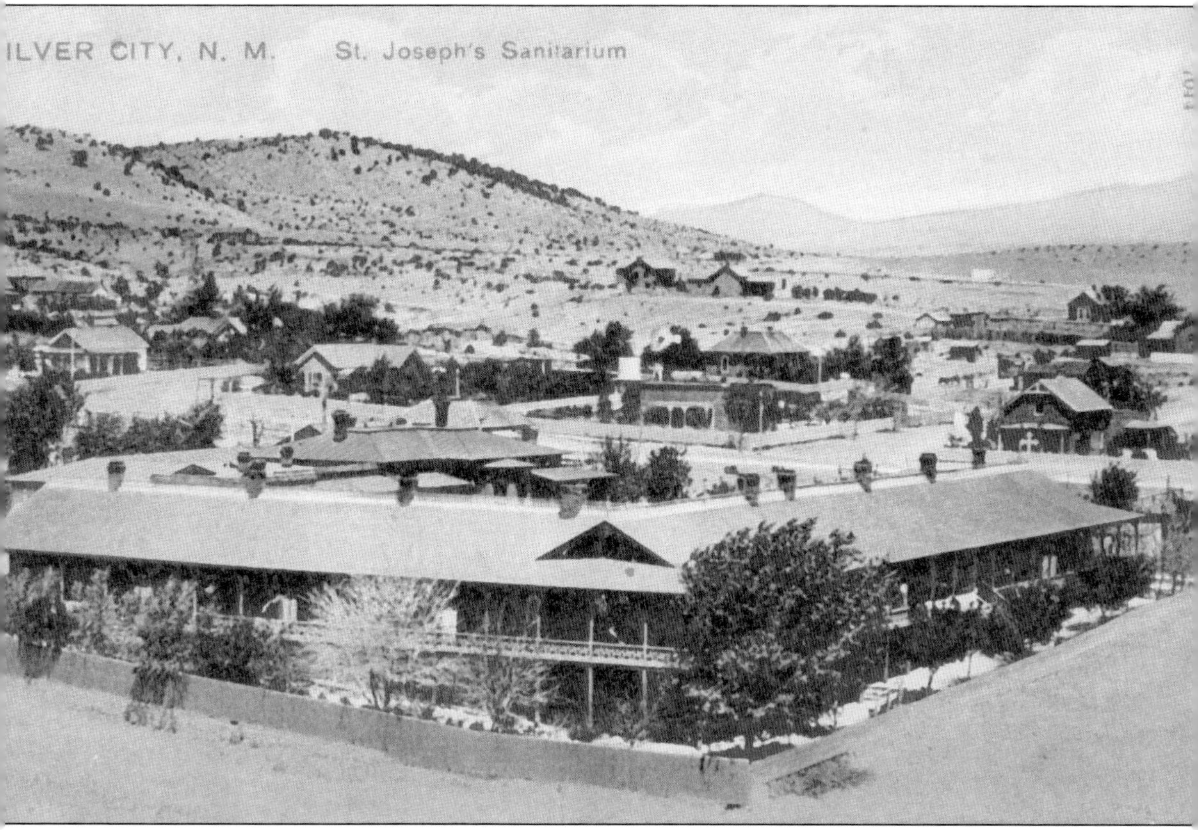

The Sisters of Mercy opened Silver City's first hospital in 1891. Eleven years later, the nuns, working with Dr. Earl S. Bullock, expanded their operation to include a sanatorium to serve the increasing number of lungers arriving daily in Silver City. The *Silver City Independent* enthusiastically reported that Dr. Bullock received inquiries from "all over the United States," meaning that the new san's "success is assured." Bullock praised the local climate, especially the lack of sandstorms that plagued other parts of the Southwest and were "positively detrimental" to lungers. Front and back doors to each patient's room improved access to Silver City's therapeutic mountain air. Sold by the 1920s, the old sanatorium is now an apartment complex known as St. Joseph's Square. (Courtesy of Jim Coad.)

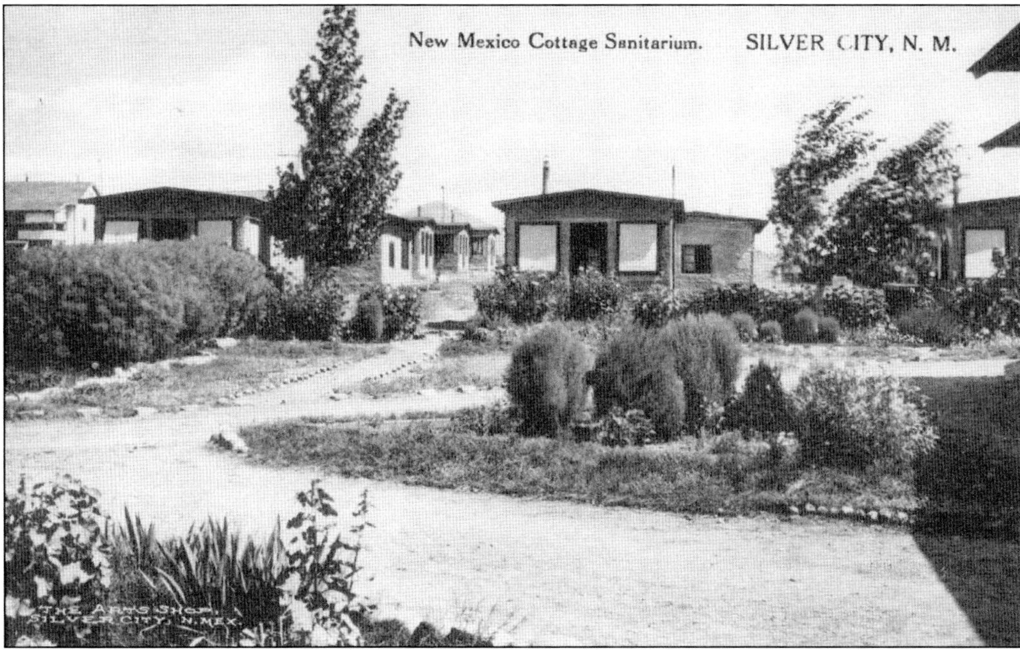

The New Mexico Cottage Sanatorium was founded in 1905 by Wayne McVeigh Wilson and Dr. Earl S. Bullock, who had formerly worked at Fort Bayard and St. Joseph's in Silver City. Starting with Founders House and 12 cottages, the institution grew to become the largest san in Silver City, with a capacity of 80 patients by 1912. A valuable asset to its community, the sanatorium purchased from grateful local suppliers "nearly every stick of wood, sack of cement, gallon of paint, [ton of] coal, [piece of] furniture, [and bit of] food," according to the *Silver City Independent*. (Both, courtesy of Jim Coad.)

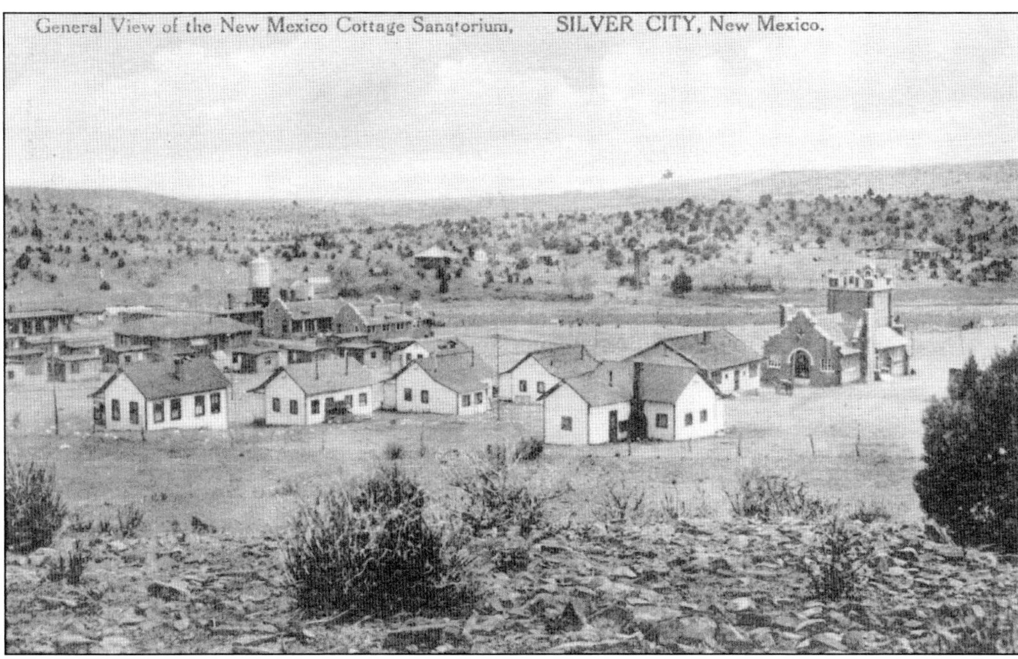

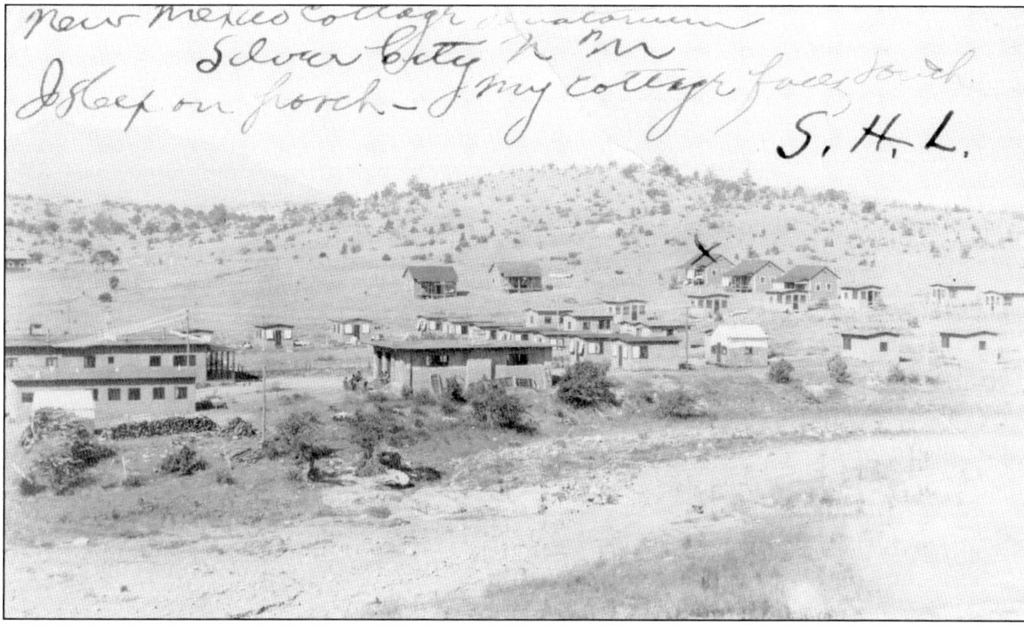
New Mexico Cottage Sanatorium
Silver City N M
I sleep on porch - x my cottage faces south.
S. H. L.

Reflecting the age group of many of their residents, cottages often resembled college dorm rooms, with pennants, photographs, and piles of books. With excellent accommodations, the Cottage Sanatorium was one of the most expensive in the state, charging up to $100 per month, equal to about $2,200 in today's money. (Above, courtesy of Nancy Tucker; below, courtesy of the Museum of New Mexico, no. 51094.)

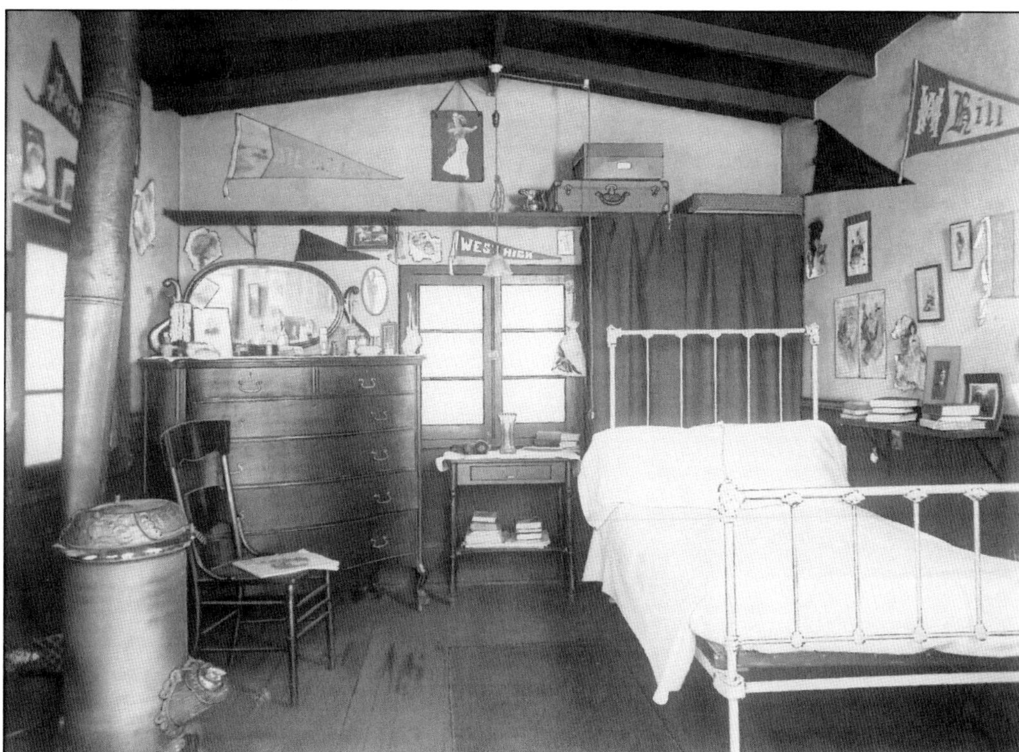

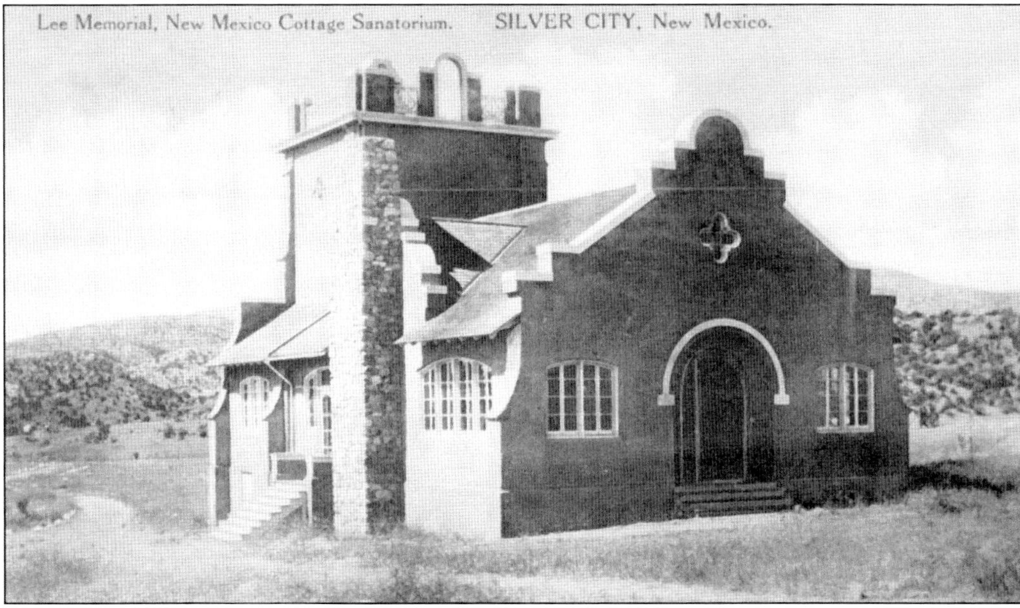

Built in 1908 and named for Aubrey Ferrell Lee, the Lee Memorial Chapel was used not only for religious services, but also for events ranging from weddings to theatrical productions. Philanthropist John Wanamaker donated $3,000 of his business fortune for the purchase of a magnificent organ for the chapel. Ironically, the chapel was destroyed by fire in 1922, the same year that Wanamaker died in Philadelphia. (Courtesy of Nancy Tucker.)

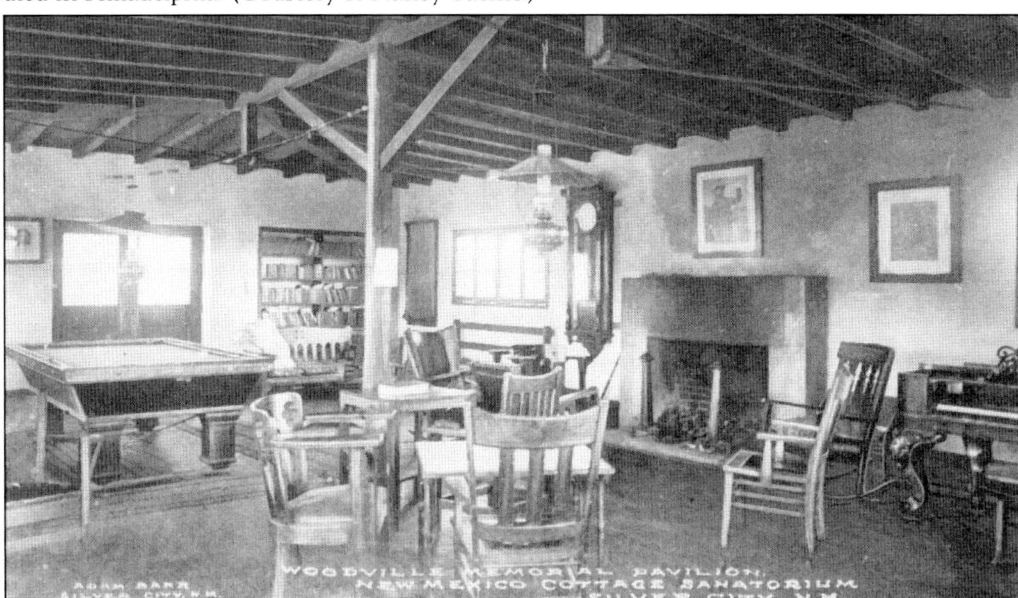

The Cottage Sanatorium, like most private sans, raised money from contributors across the country. Buildings were often named for those who gave. When Henry Woodville succumbed to TB after several years of "chasing," friends contributed funds for a building, which was named the Woodville Pavilion and Recreation Hall. Individual cottages cost $300 to construct and $150 to furnish. By 1907, forty-two cottages had been built around a central courtyard. (Courtesy of Nancy Tucker.)

The New Mexico Cottage Sanatorium closed in 1924 and was purchased by George Washington Pennington. Like so many lungers, Pennington had first come to New Mexico with only a few months to live, but he beat the odds and became a successful businessman and two-time mayor of Silver City. According to health historian Doc Campbell, at least one building, the Anne Thomson Infirmary, became a private home. Many of the old cottages were sold individually and moved into Silver City, where they can still be found today. Even without its largest san, Silver City remained one of New Mexico's communities with the highest percentage of TB patients. As late as 1951, thirty percent of all lungers in the state lived in Grant County. (Both, courtesy of Nancy Tucker.)

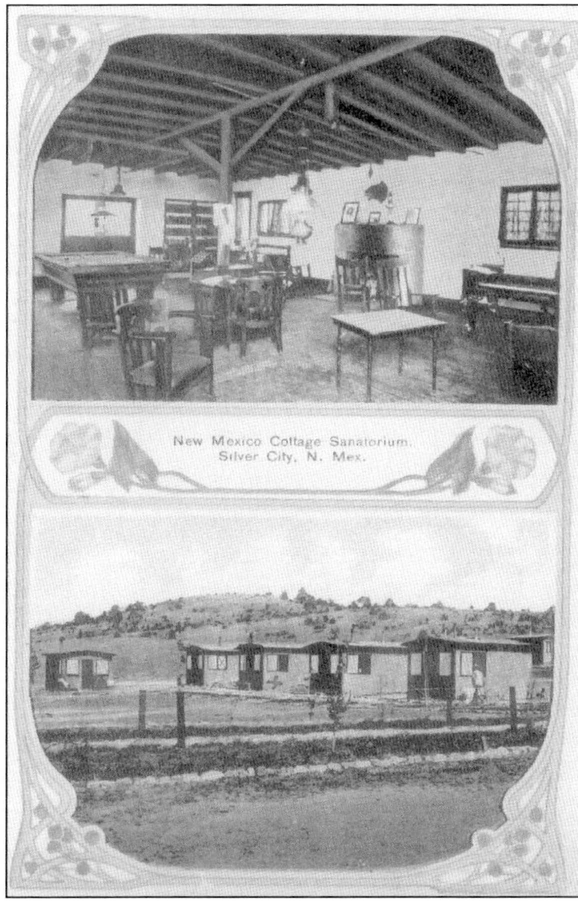

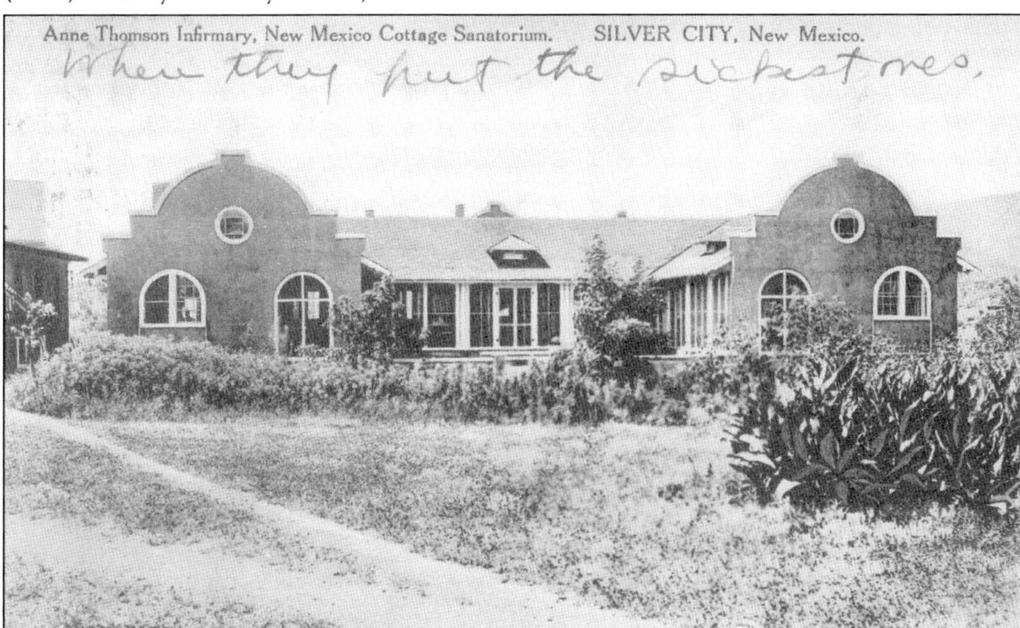

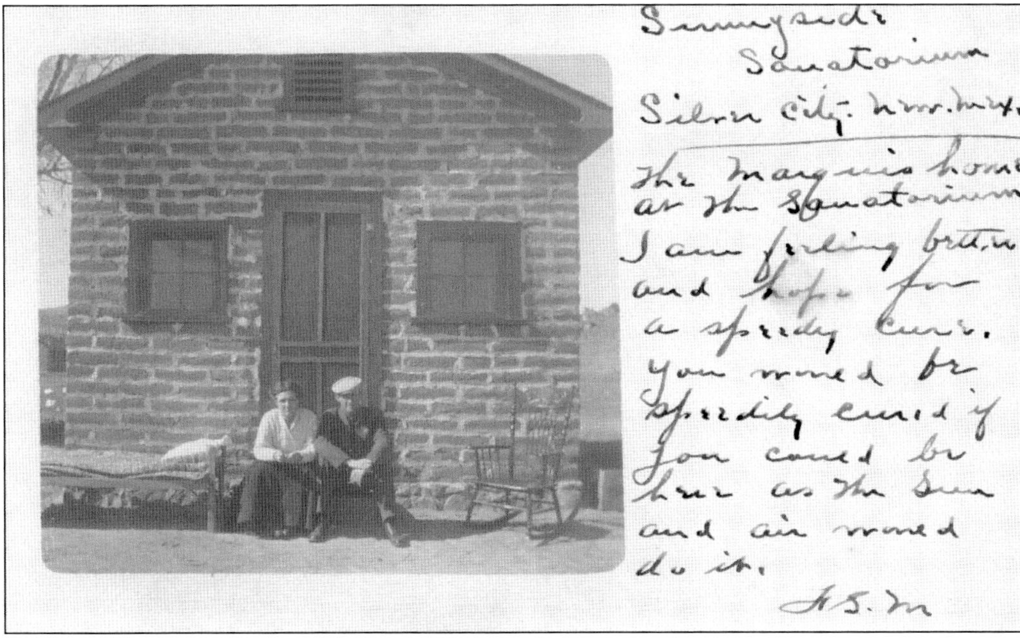
Sunnyside
Sanatorium
Silver City. New Mex.
The Marquis home
at the Sanatorium.
I am feeling better
and hope for
a speedy cure.
You would be
speedily cured if
you could be
here as the sun
and air would
do it.
H.S.M

Located on the 60-acre Woodhull Ranch north of Silver City, Sunnyside Sanatorium opened in early 1909 as a lower-priced option to the nearby New Mexico Cottage Sanatorium. Thornton Moore soon purchased the san, but then sold it to Albuquerque's Methodist san for $9,000 in 1915. Sunnyside included a large administration building, 18 one-room cottages, and several larger cottages on the property. (Courtesy of Charles Kohlass.)

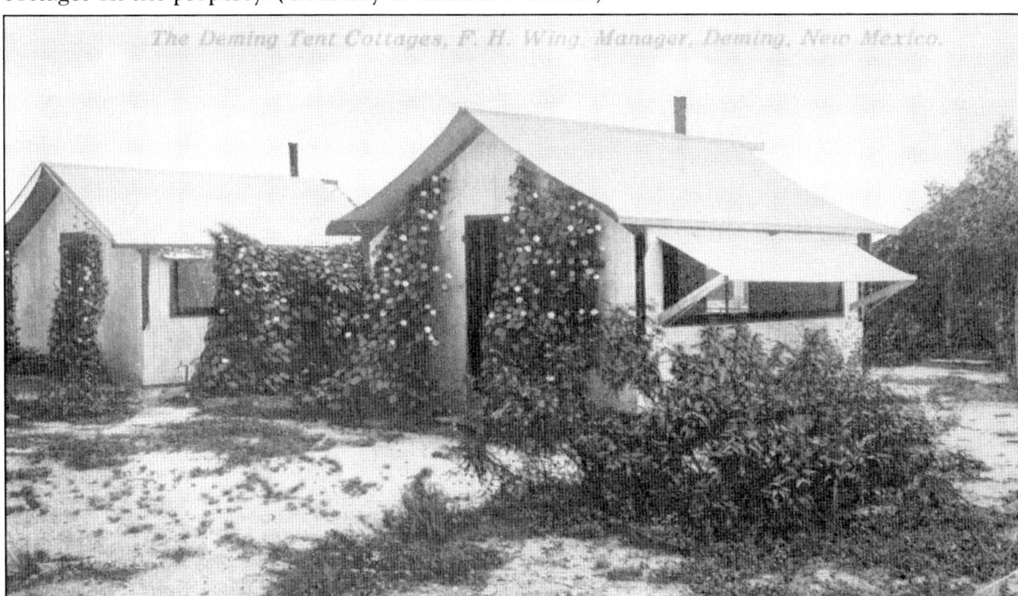
The Deming Tent Cottages, F. H. Wing, Manager, Deming, New Mexico.

In 1914, community leaders in Deming announced plans for a $50,000 sanatorium to be built on 20 acres of land southwest of town. The *Las Cruces Estrella* reported that cottages were to be built with "every possible aid to render them attractive." The san opened in 1916, with nine lungers under the care of Dr. Janet Reid, a rare female TB specialist in New Mexico. (Courtesy of Nancy Tucker.)

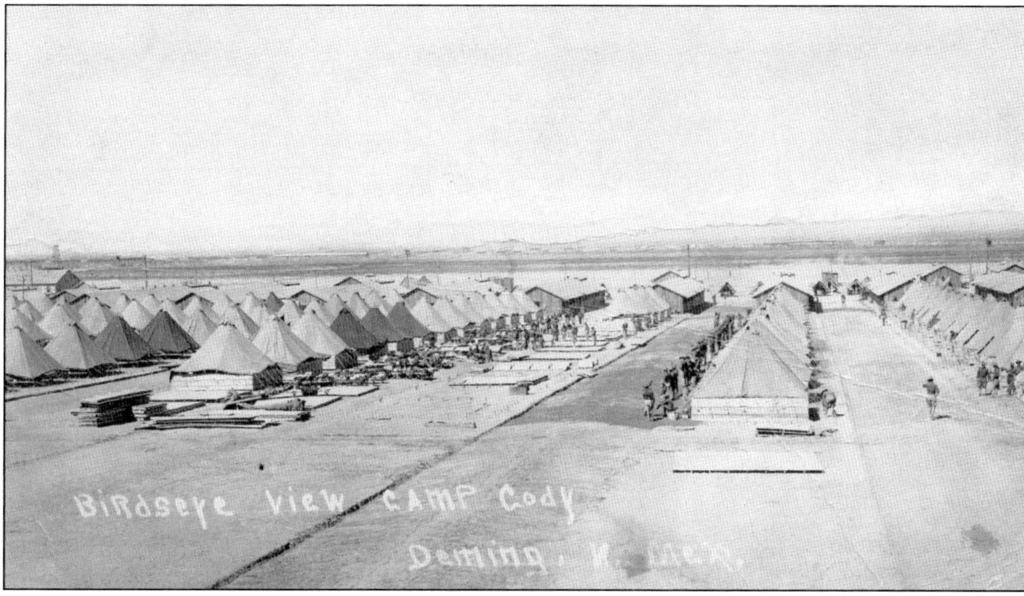

Located west of Deming, Camp Cody had been built to train soldiers during World War I. With the end of the war, the local chamber of commerce purchased the property and then sold it to the Sisters of the Holy Cross. The camp was converted into a modern san, as buildings were renovated and new structures were added at a cost of $250,000. Bishop Anthony J. Schuler dedicated the new sanatorium in 1923.

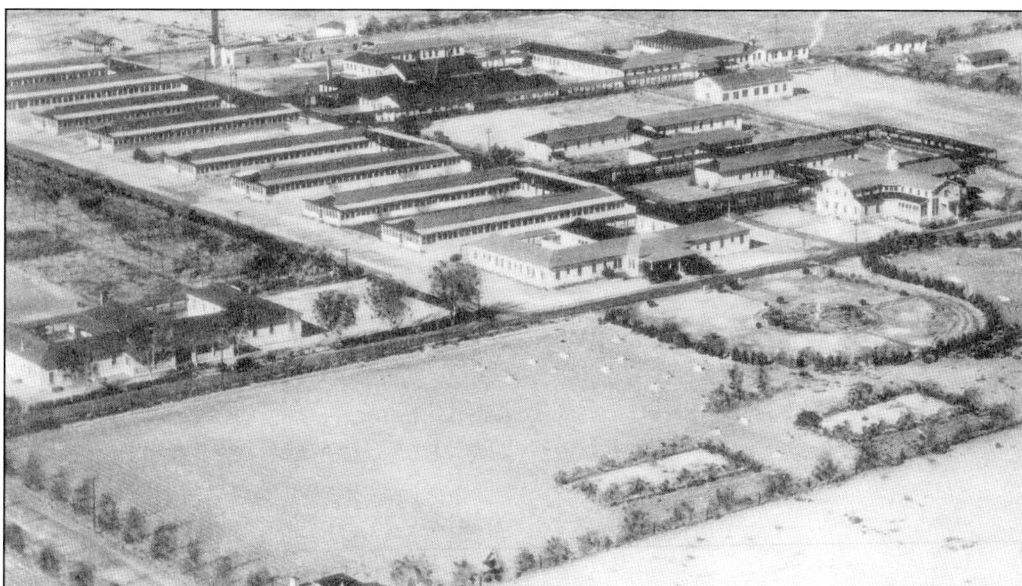

Holy Cross promoted its "99.99 percent" pure water, "not uncomfortable" summers, and "few" spring sandstorms. Eugenia Wagner of Minnesota became the san's first patient. Over the next 15 years, 1,047 patients, including many priests and nuns, followed. A female patient's sister was a Harvey Girl in Deming who worked hard to finance her sibling's medical care. Mildred Clark (the Harvey Girl) later turned to more lucrative employment, becoming New Mexico's infamous Madame Millie.

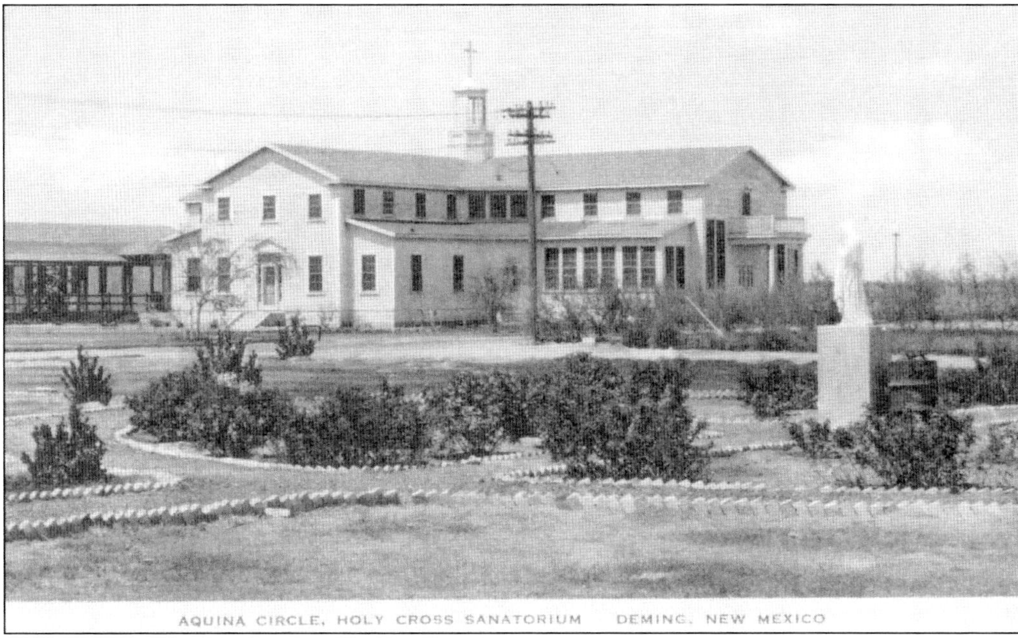
AQUINA CIRCLE, HOLY CROSS SANATORIUM DEMING, NEW MEXICO

From 1923 to 1938, a total of 65 Holy Cross nuns served at the san, including Sister Marcelle Groarke, who worked the entire 15 years. The nuns performed all sorts of labor, from caring for their patients and helping with the san's 20-cow dairy, to working in the san's fourth-class US post office. Holy Cross became as self-supporting as possible in order to cut costs for its patients and to reduce operating costs as a whole. Holy Cross even trained many of its own nurses, opening a nurse's training school in 1929 and capping its first four graduates in 1933. (Above, courtesy of Nancy Tucker; below, courtesy of Jim Coad.)

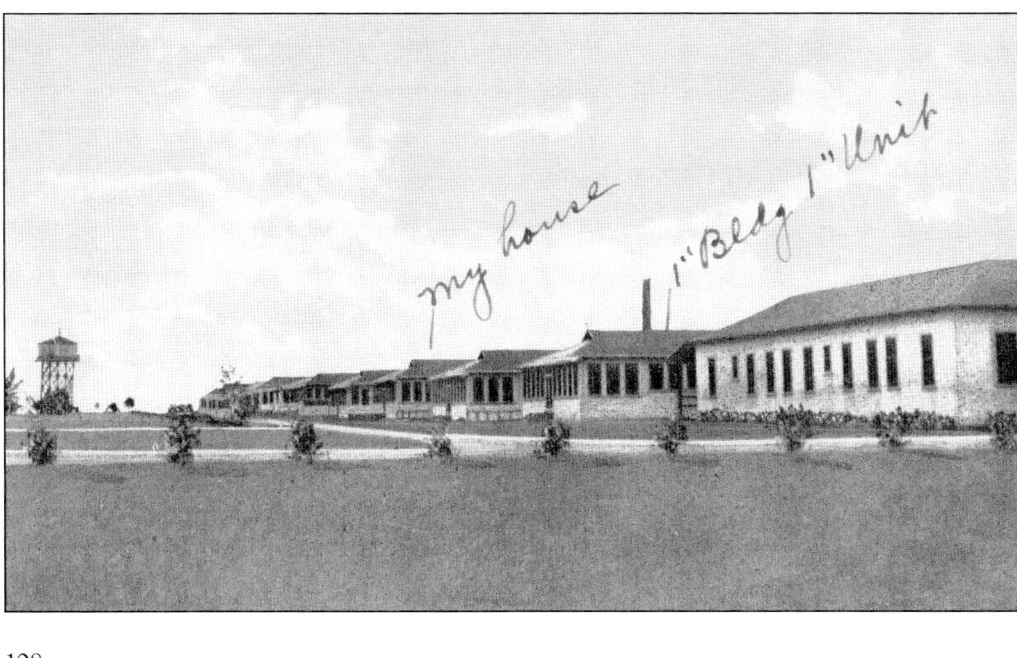
my house
1" Bldg 1" Unit

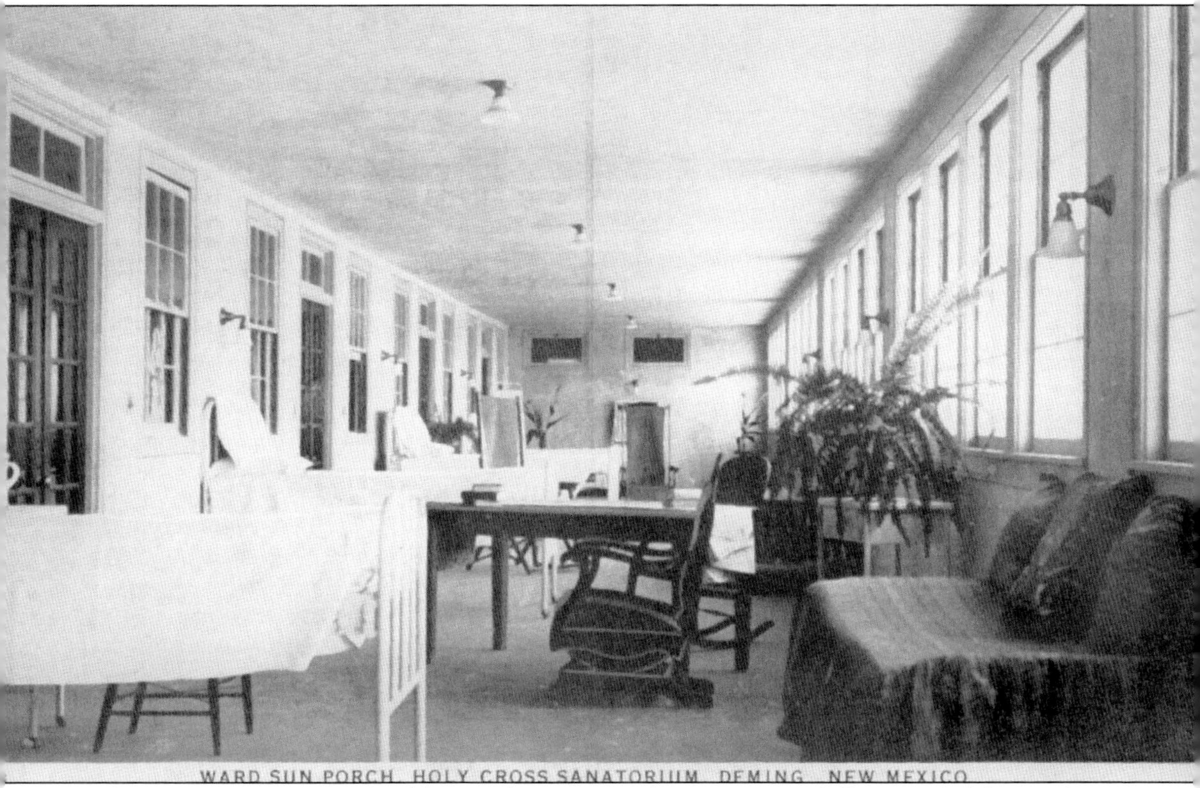

While many recovered their health at Holy Cross, 147 (or 14 percent of all patients) did not. The bodies of most of those who died were transported by train to their home states (mostly in the Midwest) for burial. Others were buried in the two-acre cemetery east of the san, starting with an Irish priest who died in 1924. The san itself began to die during the Great Depression, when too few potential patients could afford the $750 per year charge for a ward bed and too many men and women were accepted as charity patients. Heavily in debt, the sisters made the tough decision to close their san in 1938. On Sunday, March 12, 1939, a mysterious fire destroyed 13 of the san's 16 buildings—fortunately with no injuries or loss of life. When the sisters' fire insurance policy paid the balance of the san's outstanding debt, a sister proclaimed that the blaze was "God's solution to our problem." (Courtesy of Nancy Tucker.)

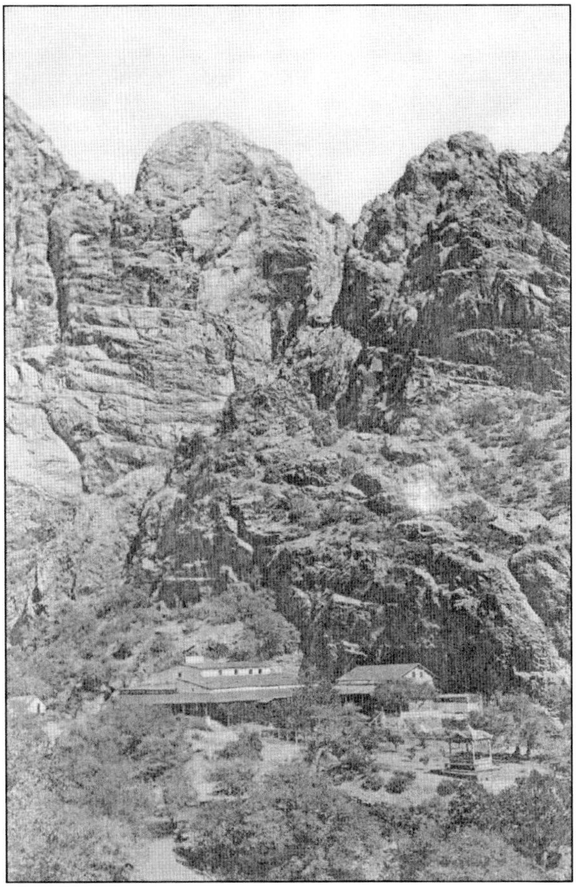

Former Confederate colonel Eugene Van Patten opened Van Patten's Mountain Camp at Dripping Springs in the Organ Mountains, east of Las Cruces, in the 1870s. The resort included 16 guest rooms, a large dining room, and a concert hall. Arriving by stagecoach, guests from El Paso and other uncomfortably warm locations often came to Van Patten's to escape the summer heat in beautiful, cool surroundings. The resort flourished for 40 years. Dr. Nathan Boyd of San Francisco bought the property in 1917, when his wife contracted TB. Converting the resort into a san, Dr. Boyd later sold the operation to Dr. T.C. Sexton of Las Cruces. It remained open until about 1925. Now abandoned, the canyon is said to be populated by the restless spirits of patients who died during the san's short history. (Left, courtesy of Nancy Tucker; below, courtesy of Jim Coad.)

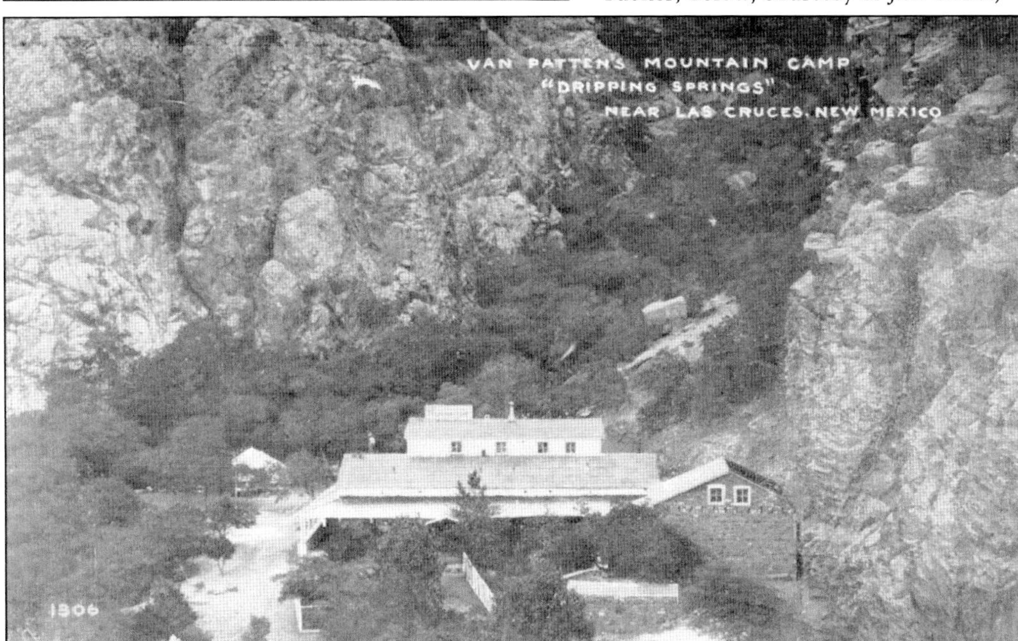
VAN PATTEN'S MOUNTAIN CAMP
"DRIPPING SPRINGS"
NEAR LAS CRUCES, NEW MEXICO
1306

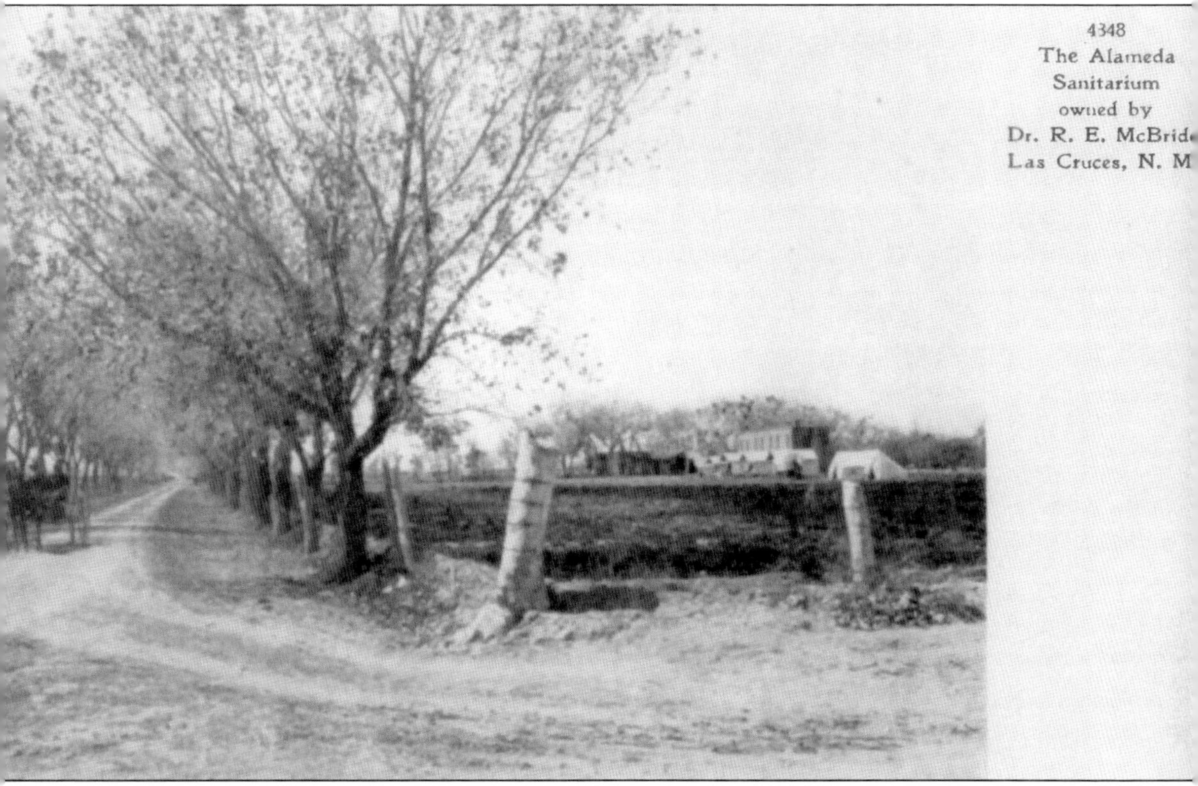
4348
The Alameda
Sanitarium
owned by
Dr. R. E. McBrid
Las Cruces, N. M

J.K. Livingston opened the Alameda Ranch Resort on a large farm north of Las Cruces in the 1890s. The resort prospered in an 11-room adobe structure, built in the Territorial style. Dr. Robert McBride, who had come to Las Cruces for his wife's health, purchased the property in 1904, creating the city's first sanatorium. A brochure promoted the "life-giving blessing" of Las Cruces' ideal air and climate. (Courtesy of Nancy Tucker.)

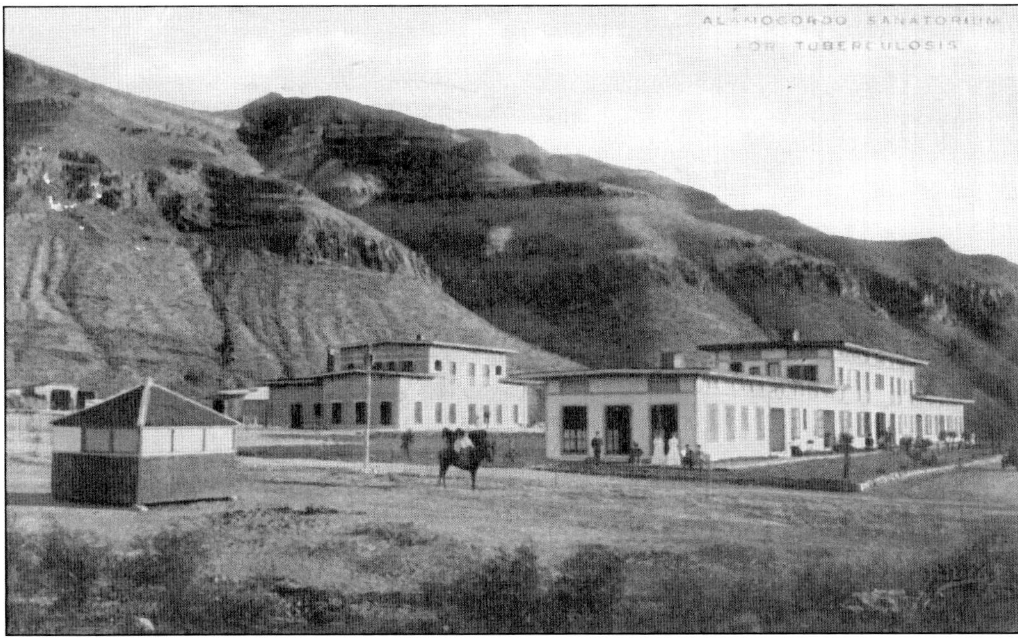
FOR TUBERCULOSIS

Aware of the positive impact of a successful san on a local economy, the Alamogordo Business Men's Club distributed promotional postcards when the 100-patient Fraternal City Sanatorium opened in 1907. The back of one postcard boasts that the new san is "not a private institution for profit but a humanitarian sanatorium where patients will receive the best of care and attention at about the actual cost of their keeping, making it the cheapest modern home in this country for those suffering with tuberculosis." Despite its name, not all relations were fraternal at the san. In 1909, its medical director, Dr. O.M. Miller, drew a revolver and shot the san's proprietor, W.A. Reid, in a dispute over money. At times known as the Alamogordo or American Cooperative Sanatorium, the property burned down about 1912, but it later reopened for several years.

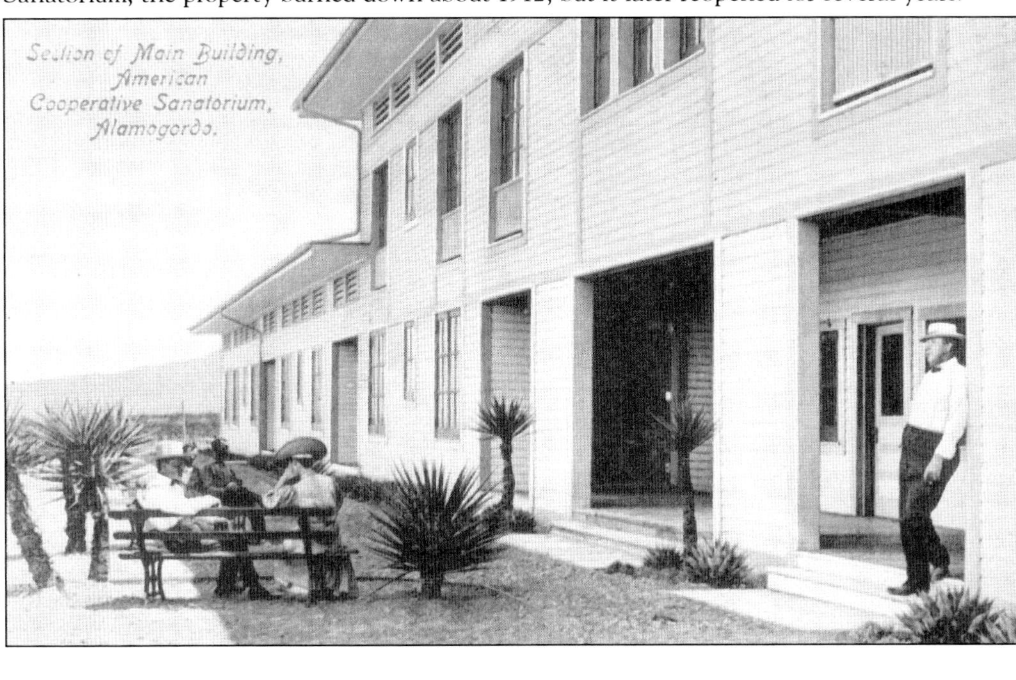
Section of Main Building,
American
Cooperative Sanatorium,
Alamogordo.

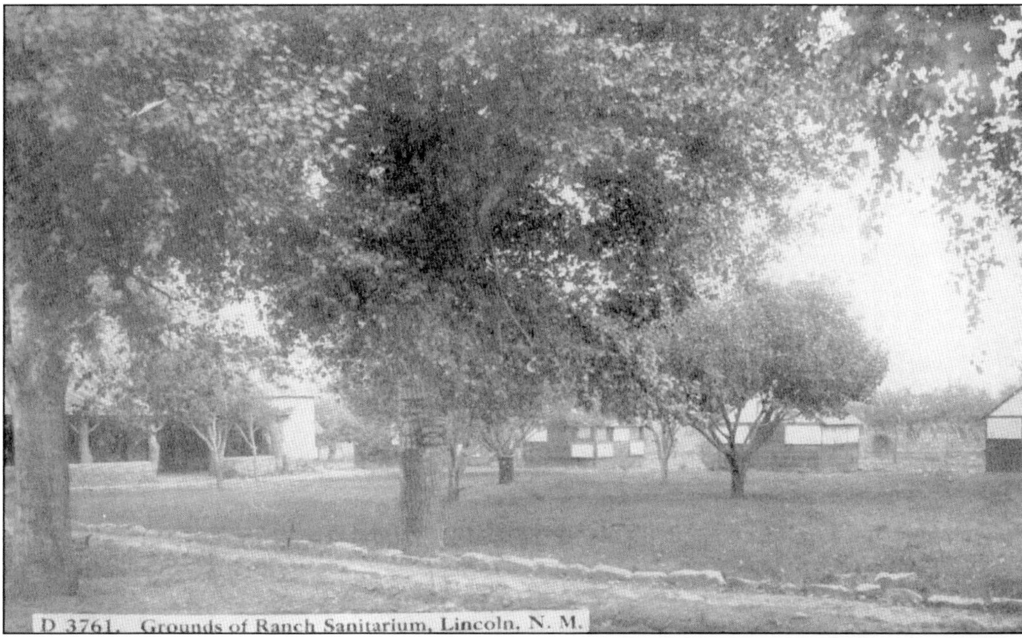

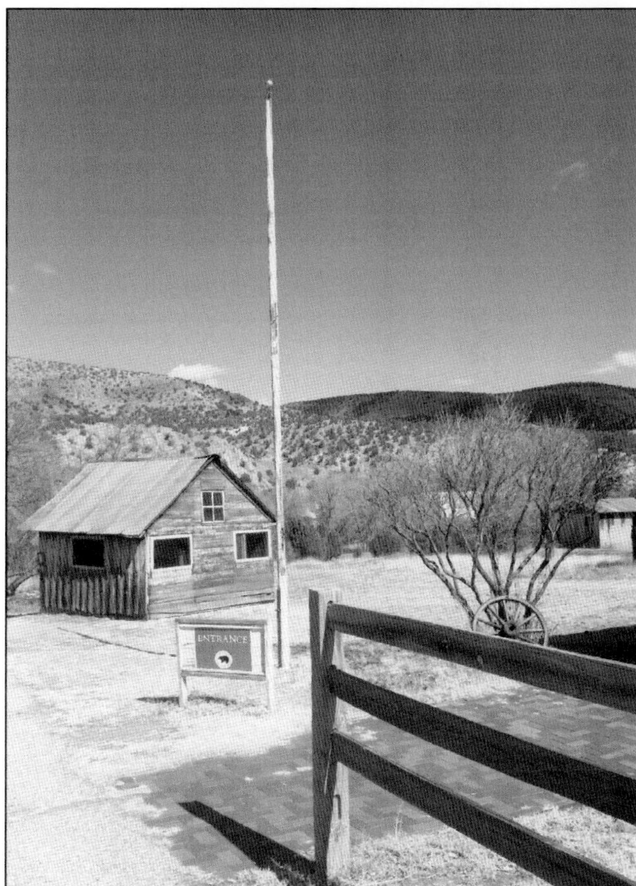

James W. Laws was a young physician in Tennessee when he fell victim to TB, "shattering all my hopes." Determined to fight the disease that had taken several relatives, Laws came to New Mexico in 1901 and recovered at Fort Stanton. Dr. Laws remained in Lincoln County, marrying Grace Austin, who had also come to New Mexico for her health. For 12 years, the couple ran a small san in Lincoln, occupying the old Ellis Store, made famous in the Lincoln County War. The doctor converted the store, established a phone line, installed Lincoln's first indoor plumbing, and built wood-frame "TB huts" (right). Grace remembered the san and its patients as "more like a family home than an institution." The san faced problems, including the "nightmare" of keeping cooks and nurses. (Above, courtesy of Nancy Tucker; right, courtesy of Gary Cozzens.)

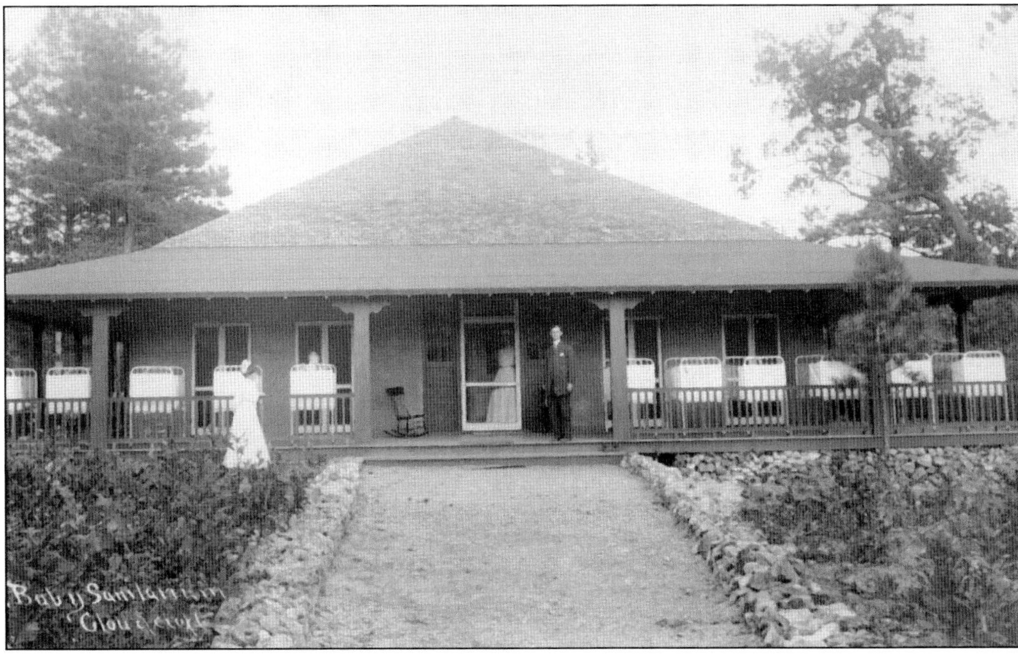

Led by Dr. Herbert E. Stevenson, a group of concerned El Paso citizens created a small sanatorium (above) for infants suffering from mostly heat-related illnesses. From 1911 to 1934, an estimated 500 babies benefited from Cloudcroft's cool summer temperatures and 8,600-foot elevation. Like most travelers to Cloudcroft, babies arrived via the famous "Cloud-Climbing Railroad" (below), the highest standard-gauge railroad in the world when it was completed in 1900. A second san for children was located on the old Baptist College campus in Alamogordo from 1913 to 1918. A third children's san opened in Silver City in 1916. (Above, courtesy of Nancy Tucker.)

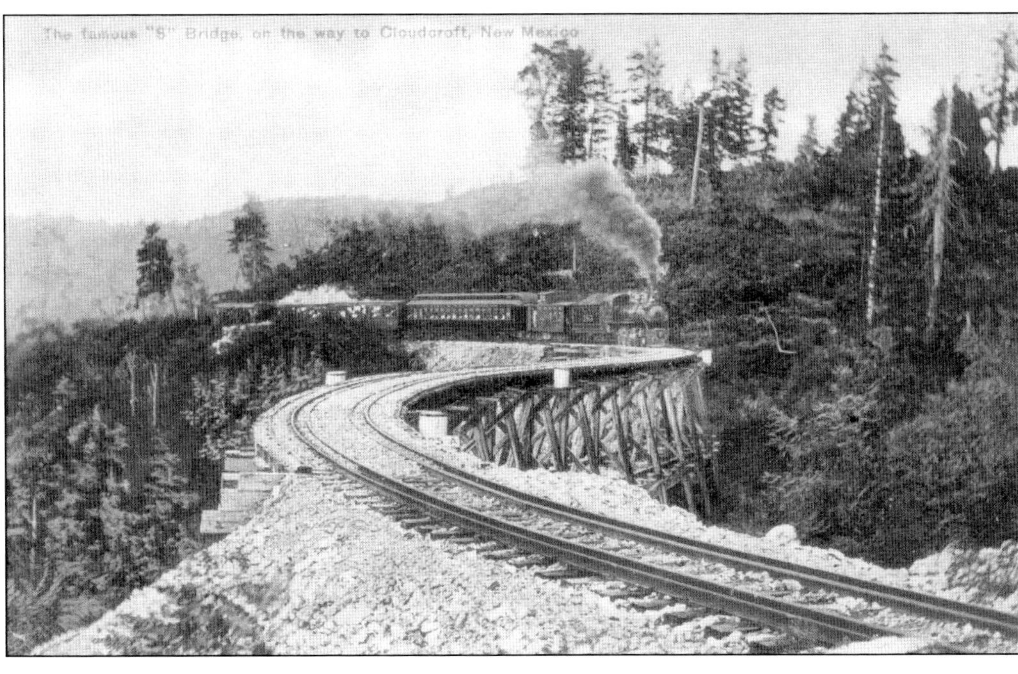
The famous "S" Bridge, on the way to Cloudcroft, New Mexico

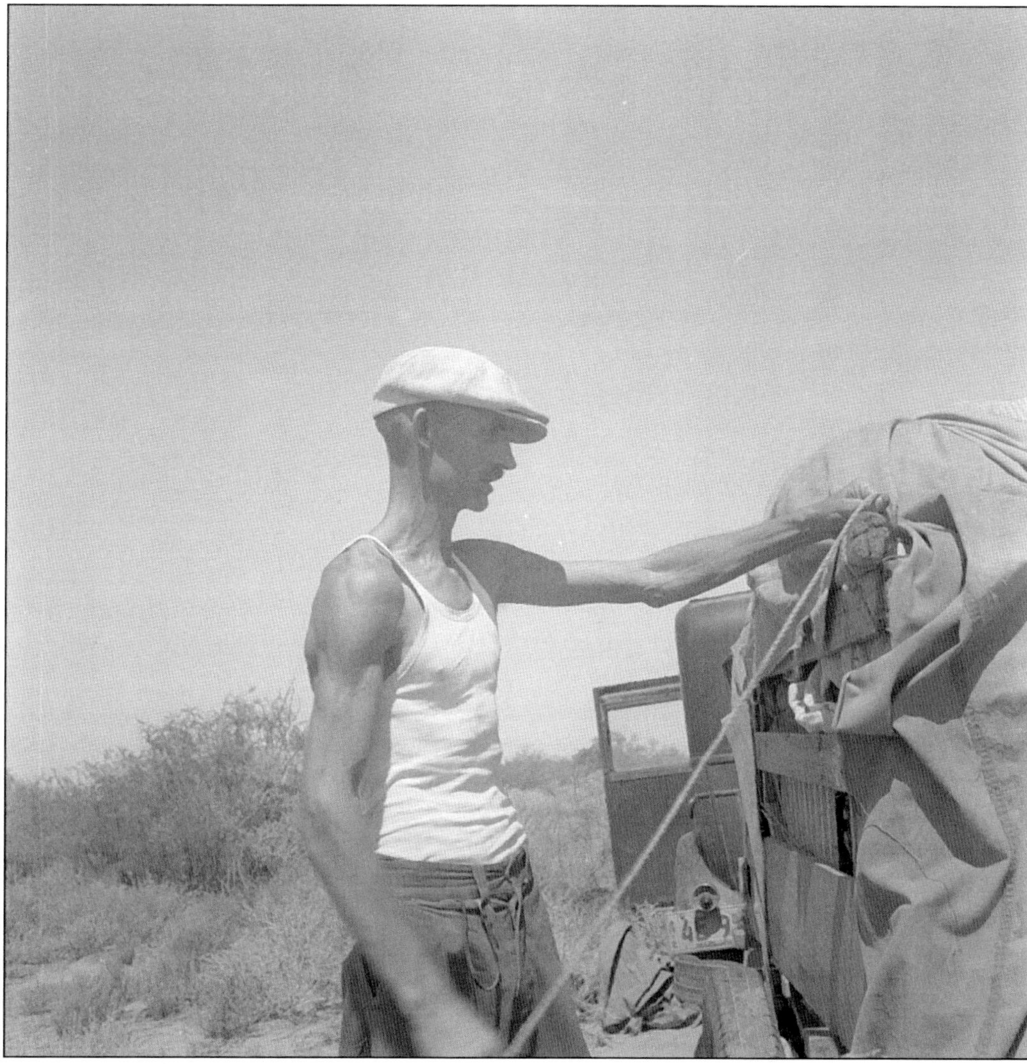

A vast wave of transient lungers had arrived in New Mexico by the early 20th century, causing a strain on local resources and complaints from healthy residents. Conditions grew worse during the Great Depression, when an estimated 50 percent of transient health-seekers applied for public aid within months of their arrivals. States like Illinois and New York were accused of shipping off health-seekers with "charity train tickets" that cost home institutions far less than the years of continuous assistance these patients often required. Patients who paid their own fares often spent their last dollars on their tickets to New Mexico, leaving nothing for their care after they arrived. Once in New Mexico, these newcomers were seen as a danger to state residents who came in contact with them at filling stations, restaurants, and other public places. New Mexicans had stressed the need for a public san to assist the poor—and to protect state residents—as early as 1917. Farm Security Administration photographer Dorothea Lange captured this stranded tubercular father of nine in mid-1936. (Courtesy of the Library of Congress.)

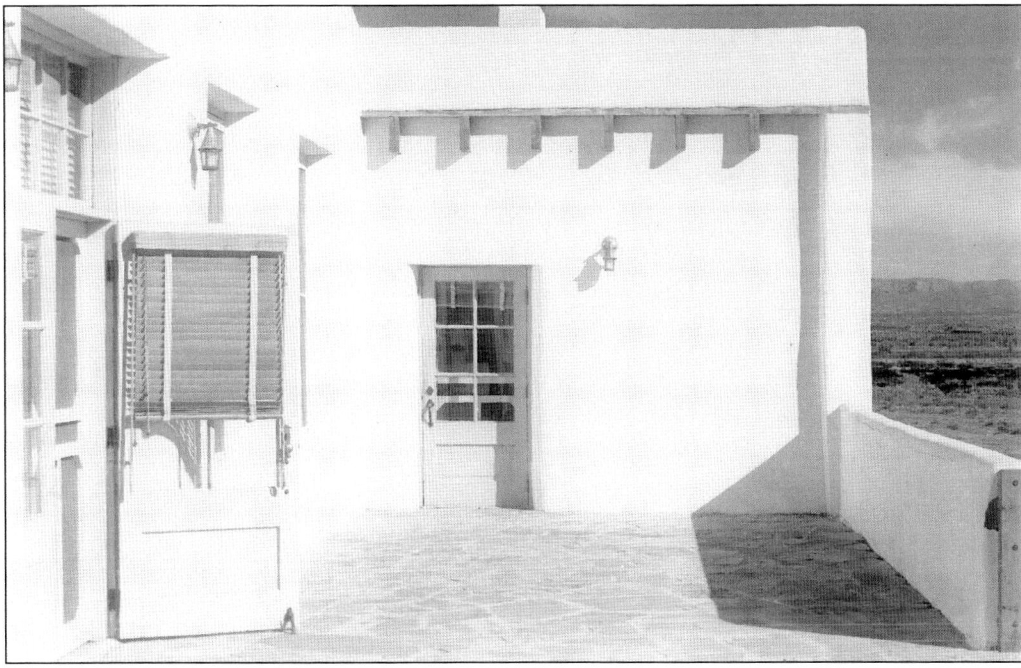

A public san, operated by the state Department of Public Welfare, was finally opened in Escondida, just north of Socorro, in 1937. The site had formerly served as CCC and transient labor camps. With new buildings erected by the WPA, the san's only requirements for admission was that a patient be a state citizen for at least a year and be unable to afford a private sanatorium. Most patients were native New Mexicans; two-thirds were Hispanic, reflecting how much TB had spread within the state. By 1940, the patient population had grown to 86. Conditions deteriorated by the mid-1950s, when patient complaints caused the firing of 50 employees and the "desertion" of 21 patients in a two-month period. The entire facility closed in mid-1957, with all remaining patients transferred to Fort Stanton. (Both, courtesy of the Socorro Historical Society.)

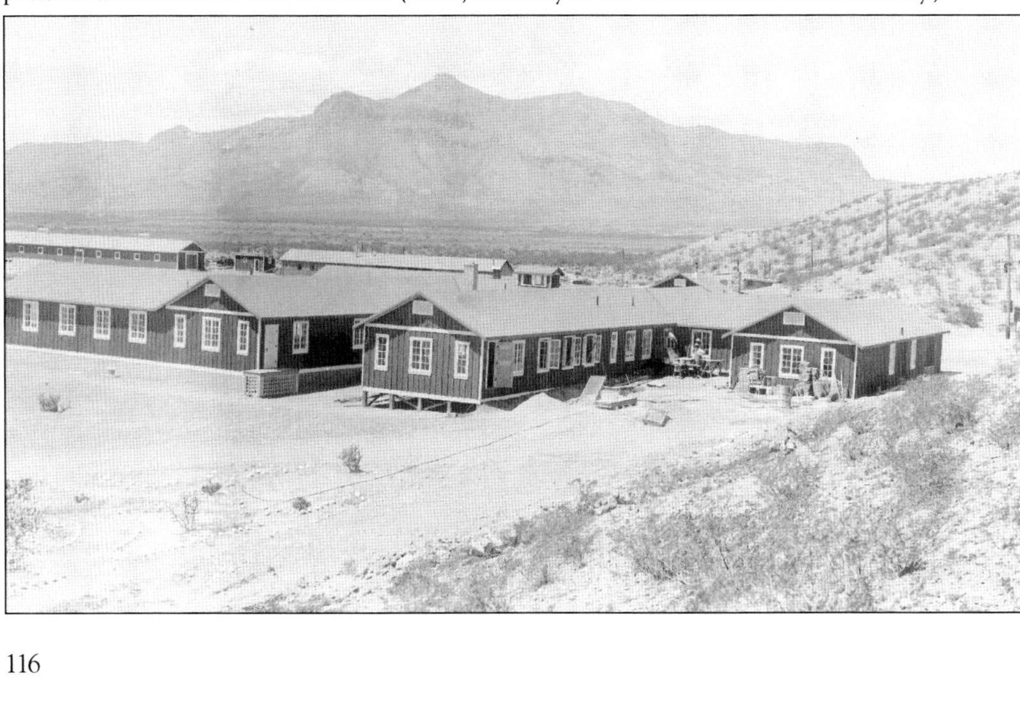

Nine

Successes and Failures

How successful were New Mexico's sanatoriums in helping to cure, or at least alleviate, the misery of tuberculosis? It appears that the odds of a health-seeker's recovery increased considerably if a person (1) came to New Mexico at an early stage of his disease, (2) had the patience and discipline to rest consistently, (3) maintained a positive attitude, (4) followed the instructions of a reliable TB specialist, and (5) could afford a good san. To paraphrase Dr. LeRoy Peters, patients bought good health care like they bought Packards, Pierces, and other good cars of their day. Unfairly, the color of recovery was largely green.

The fortunate health-seekers who recovered from TB often went home to the states they had come from. Other recovered lungers opted to stay in the Southwest, frequently making major contributions to the region. Many, like John Gaw Meem, are mentioned earlier in this book. An extended list includes Sen. Bronson Cutting, Sen. Clinton P. Anderson, New Mexico first lady Carrie Tingley, Little Theater director Kathryn O'Connor, artists Gerald Cassidy and Will Shuster, authors Alice Corbin Henderson and D.H. Lawrence, and historian Frances V. Scholes.

But, while many conquered their disease, thousands of others did not. What was true of lungers in the rest of the country was also true in New Mexico: an estimated 25 percent died in hospitals; of those who were released, 50 percent died within five years. Lacking discipline, hope, or funds, many lungers left for home prematurely. In the words of the main character in Fred Rothermell's novel *A Preface to Death* (1932), living in a san was like living in "a cell without walls . . . waiting for execution." Predictably, Vondorn's execution day arrived after he prematurely fled his fictional "Rainbow Sanitarium."

Just as Vondorn lost hope in the sanatorium cure, many New Mexicans lost their earlier enthusiasm for sanatoriums. A backlash began early in the 20th century, as more and more people developed a fear of TB and its spread within the local population. Many boardinghouses, stores, and hotels that had earlier welcomed lungers eventually refused to do business with them.

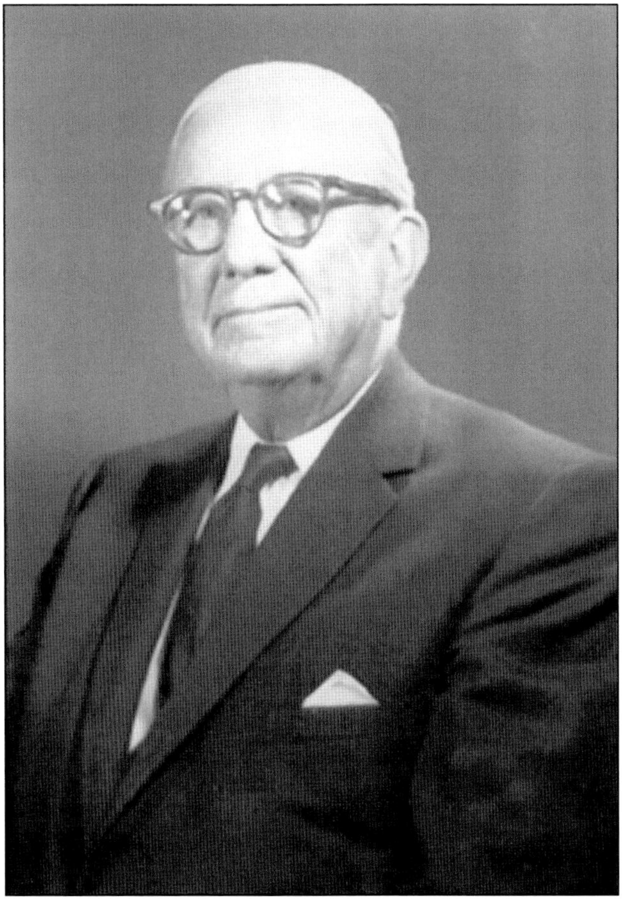

Many of New Mexico's most famous physicians first came to the Southwest as TB patients. The stellar list includes Drs. Robert O. Brown, William T. Brown, Earl Bullock, Carl Gellenthien, Frank Mera, Carl Mulky, LeRoy Peters, Abraham Shortle, and William Randolph Lovelace. Lovelace (left) had just graduated from medical school in 1905 when he was diagnosed with TB. First serving as a railroad physician in Sunnyside (now Fort Sumner), Lovelace moved to Albuquerque in 1913, where he served on the staffs of the Presbyterian, Methodist, and St. Joseph sans. By 1919, Lovelace and another former lunger, Dr. Edgar T. Lassetter, created a group practice modeled after the Mayo Clinic in Minnesota. By 1947, the Lovelace Clinic (below) had expanded into a modern research hospital. It still functions (on St. Joseph's original hospital site) as one of Albuquerque's two major medical centers. (Left, courtesy of the Lovelace Health System.)

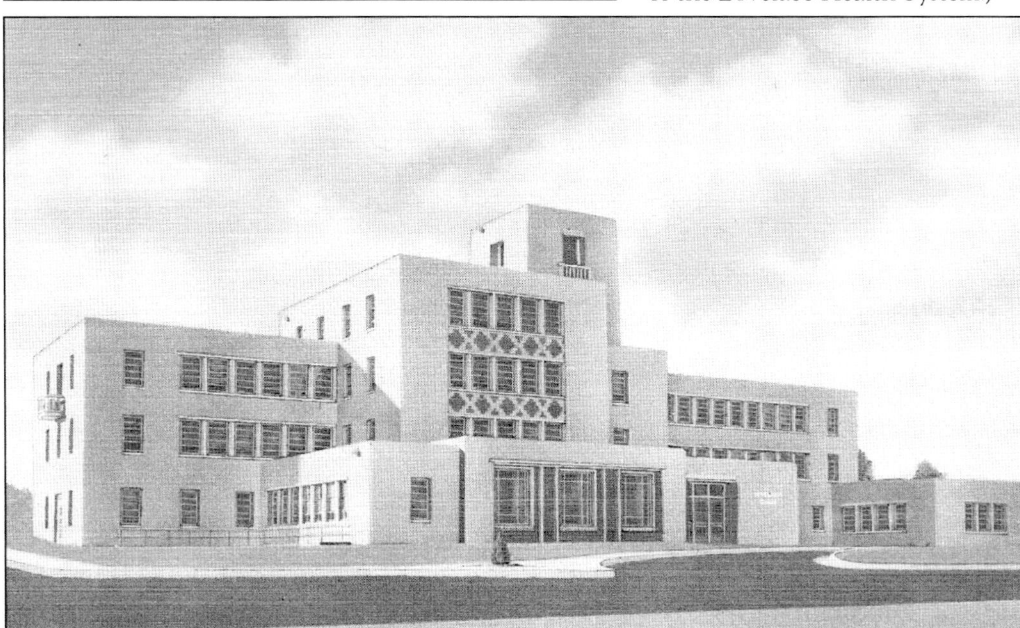

In 1910, Carrie Wooster (right) was en route by train from her native Ohio to Arizona to seek a cure for her TB. Carrie was so ill by the time she reached Albuquerque that she stopped to receive immediate medical attention. Instead of continuing on, Carrie chose to stay in New Mexico. Her fiancé, Clyde Tingley, soon joined her; they were married on April 21, 1911. Once Carrie recovered, Clyde (seen below, to her right) entered politics, rising to become the governor of New Mexico (1935–1939). The couple did everything in their power to improve conditions for patients with TB. Carrie often visited the sans, showering patients with gifts. The Tingleys' greatest contribution to TB care in New Mexico was their support for the creation of a public sanatorium, which opened in Escondido in 1937. (Right, courtesy of the Museum of New Mexico; below, courtesy of the Albuquerque Museum, PA1986-004-096.)

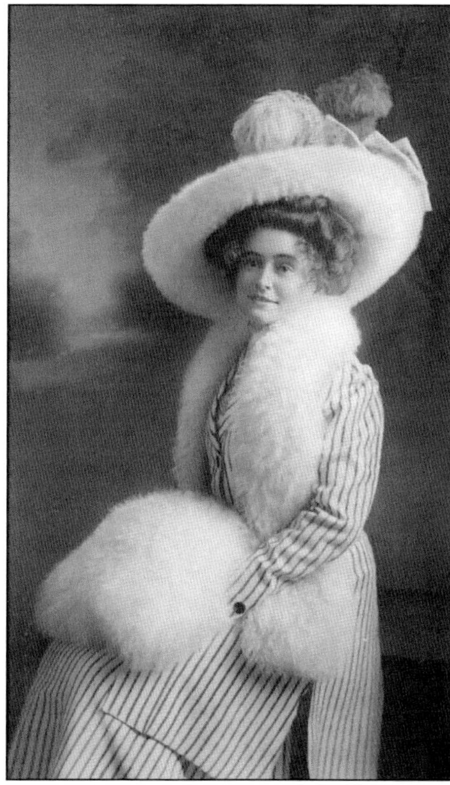

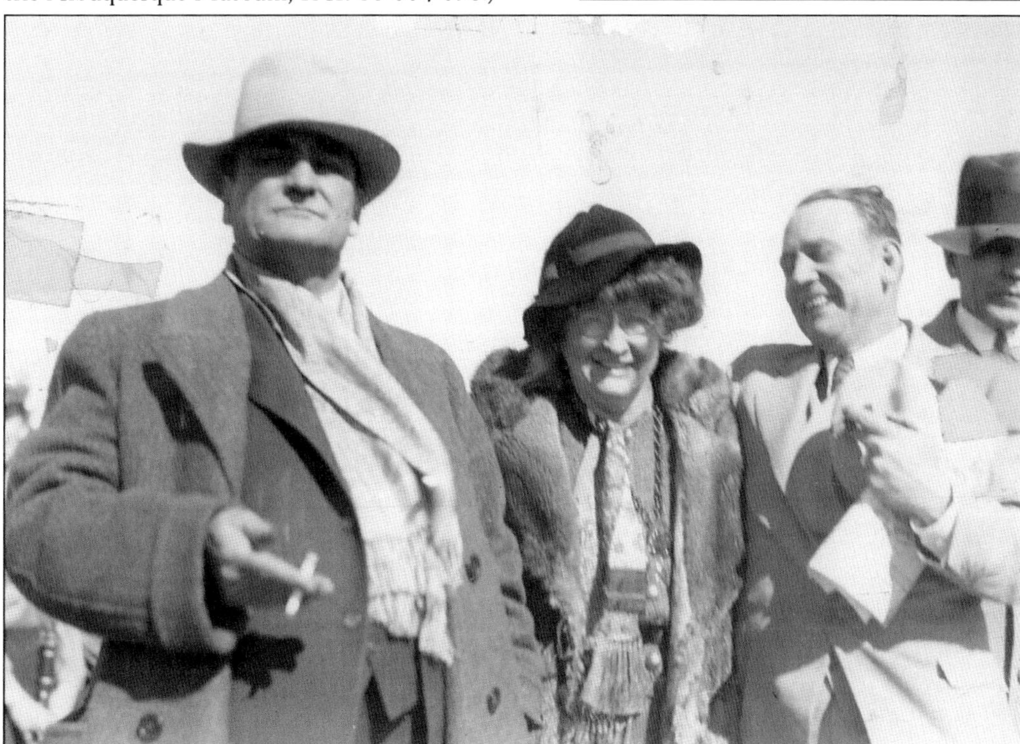

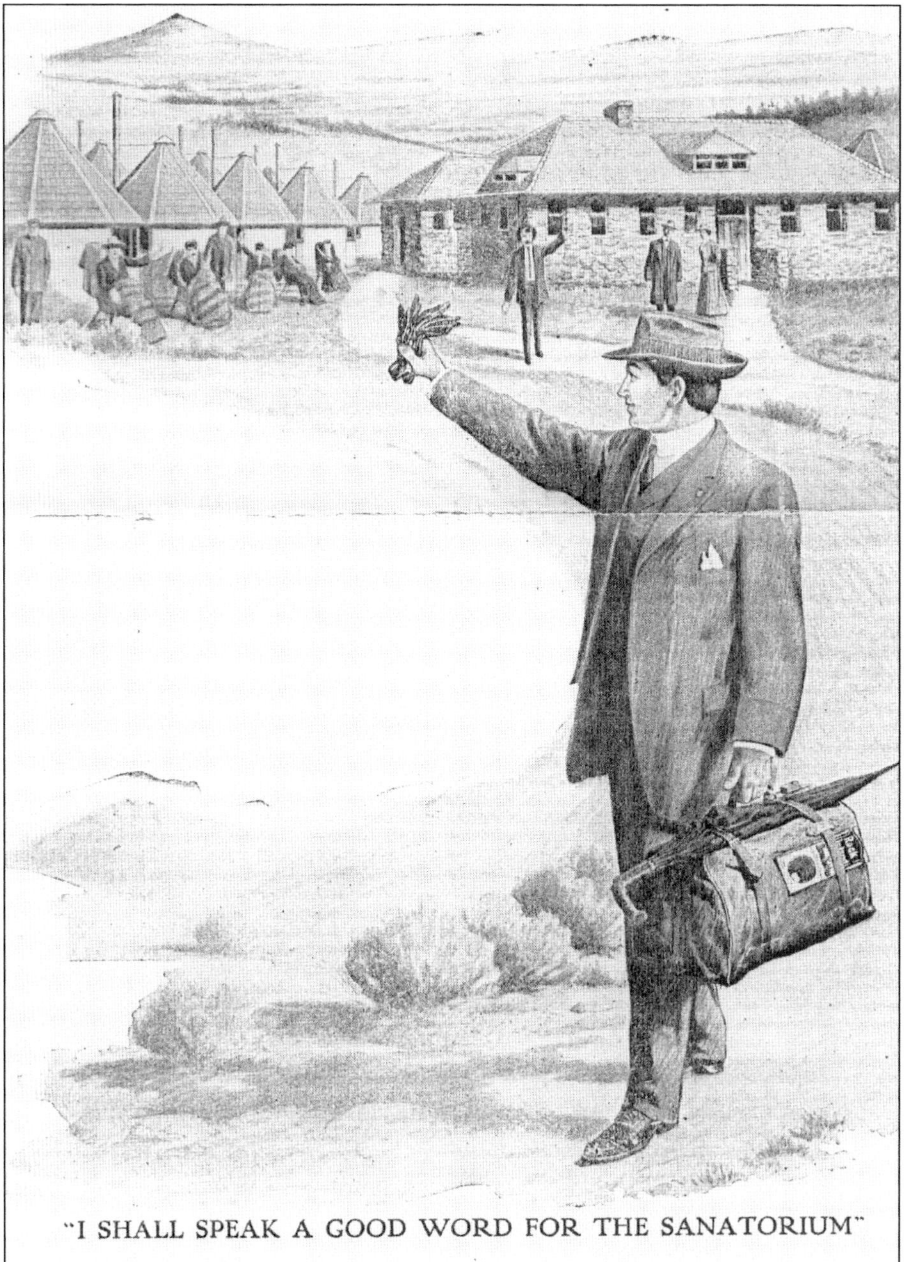

Lungers reentered the workforce as their health improved, or as the source of their funding dried up, especially during the Great Depression. While some returned to work prematurely, others thrived in employment, if only on a part-time basis. Some operated businesses from their cottages. Dick Corwine sold everything from magazines to Indian pottery and even made deliveries from his cottage at Presbyterian. Those who were ready for regular jobs were helped by Albuquerque clothes merchant Harry Spitzer, who fit each of them with a new set of clothes. Despite such encouragement, lungers often faced discrimination in the workplace and criticism from workers who competed for the same scarce jobs. As one labor leader said of Albuquerque, "Between the Mexicans and the lungers, conditions are frightful." (Courtesy of Presbyterian Healthcare Services.)

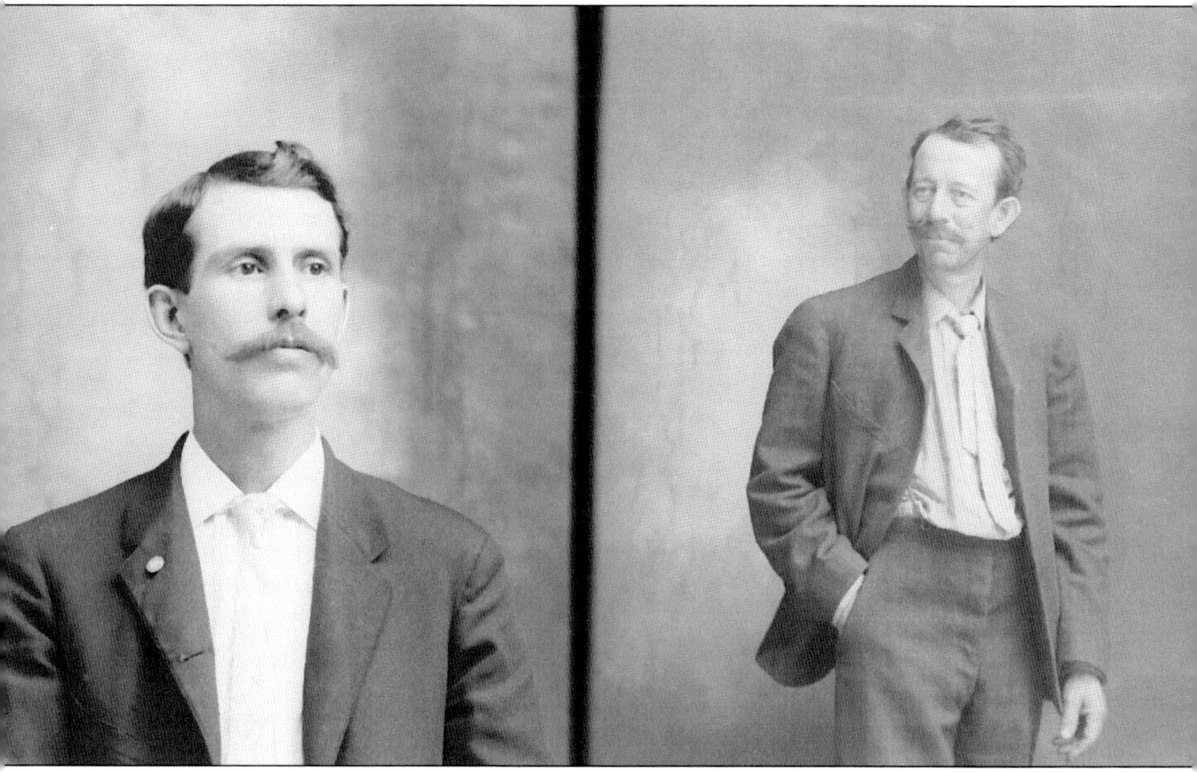

A Harvard graduate, William Henry Cobb moved to Albuquerque with a seemingly mild case of TB in 1889. He opened a photography studio and met Eddie Ross, a fellow photographer and the daughter of Edmund G. Ross, a New Mexico territorial governor. The couple married and worked together to make their studio a great success. The Cobbs photographed many men and women, including themselves. An early photograph of Cobb (left) contrasts sharply with a later image (right), when his TB had taken a heavy toll on his health. Few photographs better reflect the devastating effect of tuberculosis. Cobb died of the disease in 1909. (Courtesy of the Albuquerque Museum, PA2011-003-022.)

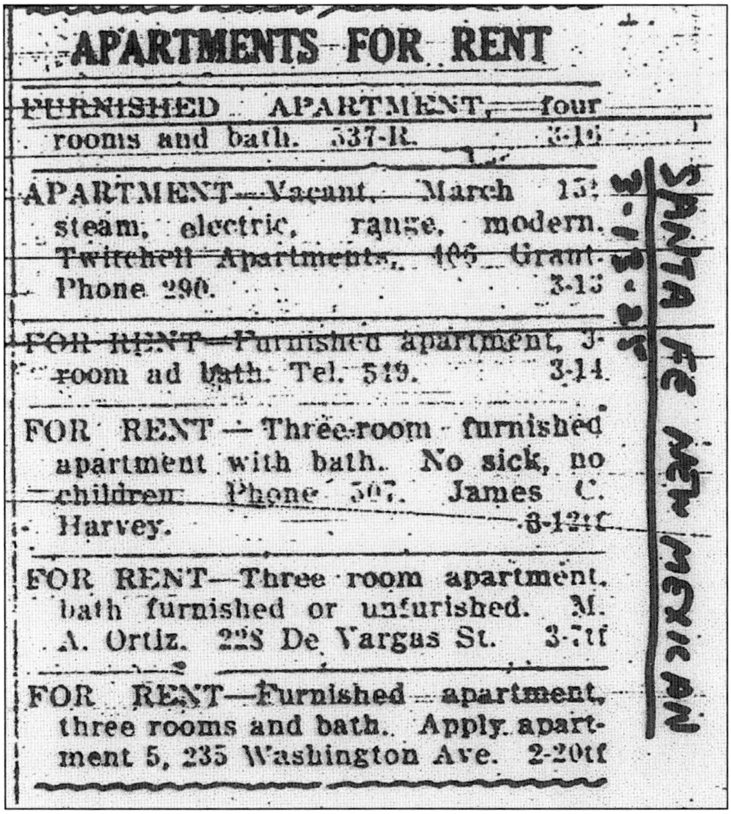

APARTMENTS FOR RENT

FURNISHED APARTMENT, four rooms and bath. 537-R. 3-16

APARTMENT—Vacant, March 13; steam, electric, range, modern. Twitchell Apartments, 106 Grant. Phone 290. 3-13

FOR RENT—Furnished apartment, 3-room ad bath. Tel. 519. 3-14

FOR RENT — Three-room furnished apartment with bath. No sick, no children. Phone 507. James C. Harvey. 3-12tf

FOR RENT—Three room apartment, bath furnished or unfurished. M. A. Ortiz. 228 De Vargas St. 3-7tf

FOR RENT—Furnished apartment, three rooms and bath. Apply apartment 5, 235 Washington Ave. 2-20tf

SANTA FE NEW MEXICAN

Many agreed with an Albuquerque resident who suspected that lungers lurked "in every block, living without regulation of any kind." When someone suggested placing placards in front of homes where lungers lived, observers countered that it would be easier to place signs at houses without lungers. As early as 1905, newspaper advertisements used the code words "no sick" to warn lungers that they were not welcome to rent certain properties.

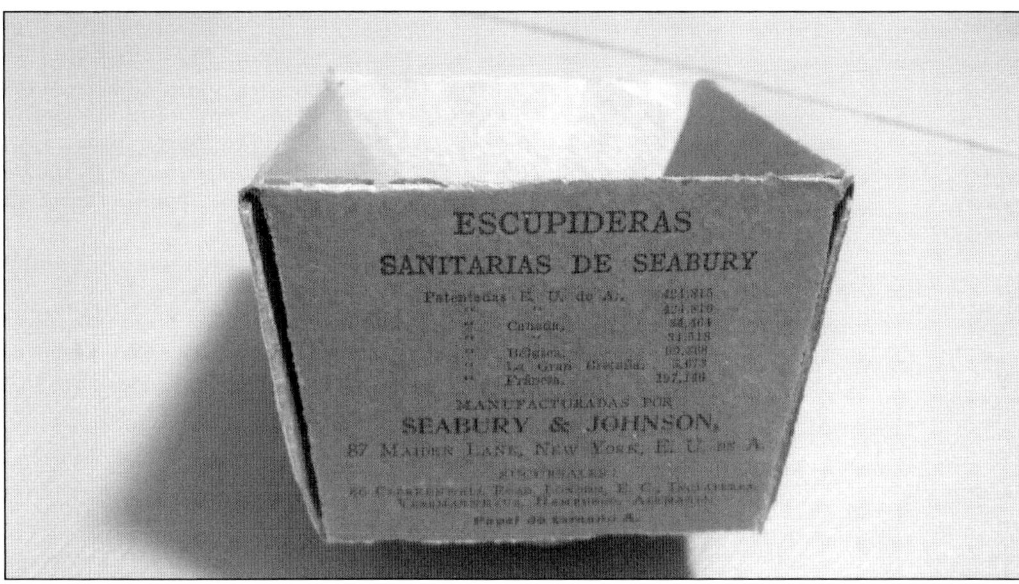

Sans urged their patients to use cardboard spitting cups, often supplying these cups and collecting them for burning in incinerators each evening. But some lungers refused to conform. TB specialists like Albuquerque's Dr. Joseph S. Cipes criticized lungers who "come down into town and . . . even if they do know better, they are ashamed to use their pocket cuspidors and so they expectorate on the streets. That's bad for the town."

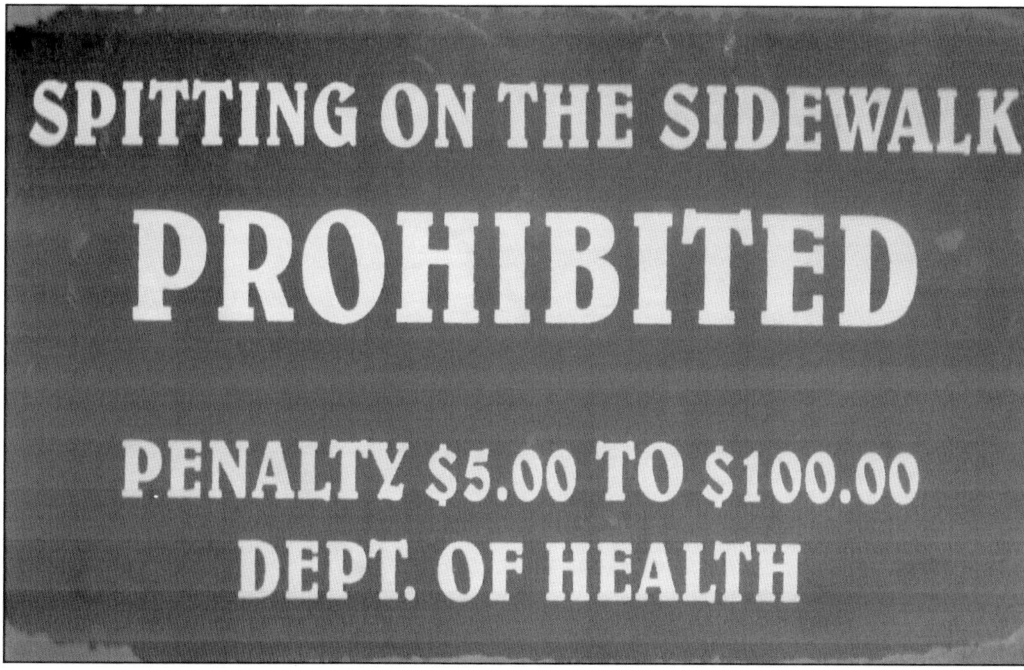

Communities across the United States passed anti-spitting ordinances in the most consistent attempt to limit the spread of tuberculosis among their citizens. Albuquerque had passed such an ordinance by 1898. Other communities in New Mexico followed suit. While most lungers obeyed these rules, some did not, causing resentment among residents. In 1901, the *Santa Fe New Mexican* wrote an indignant editorial entitled "A Filthy Habit." The newspaper criticized lungers for this "vile practice," whose ban was said to be broken 100 times a day. The territorial legislature prohibited spitting in all public places and "by-ways" throughout New Mexico in 1907.

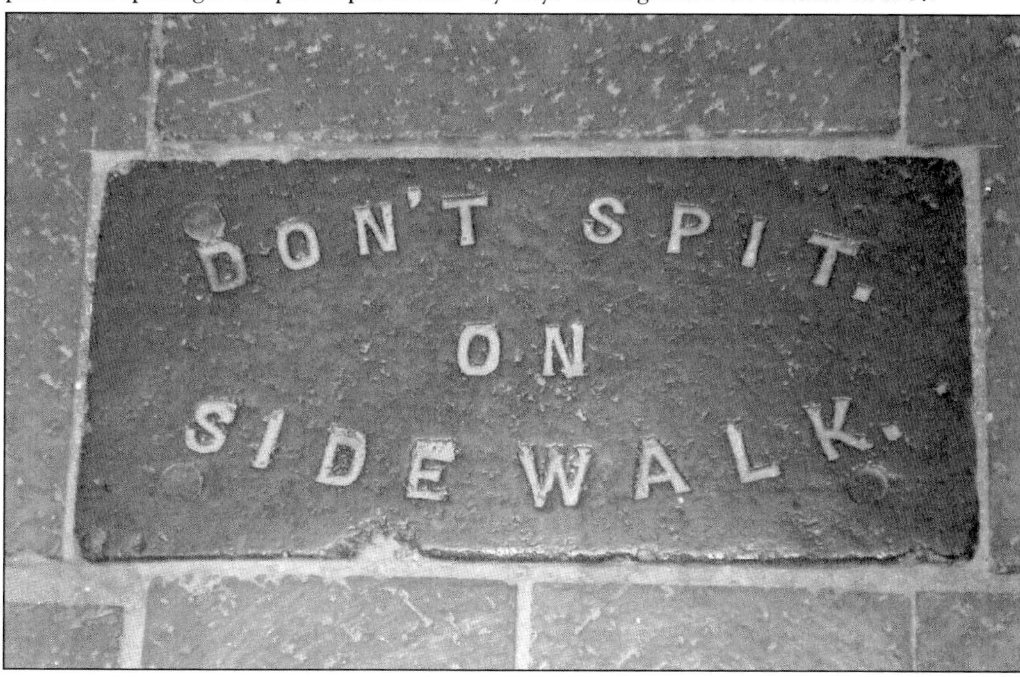

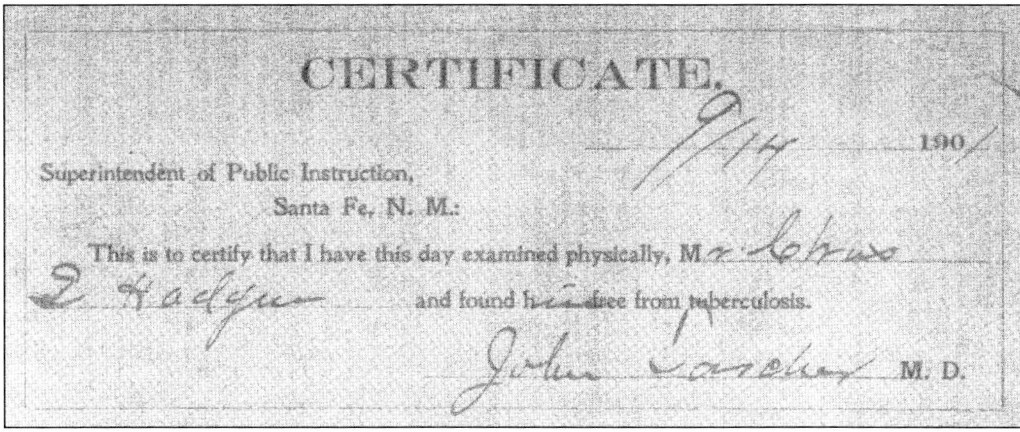

CERTIFICATE.

9/14 1901

Superintendent of Public Instruction,
Santa Fe, N. M.:

This is to certify that I have this day examined physically, M[illegible] [illegible] and found h[illegible] free from tuberculosis.

John [illegible] M. D.

Fear of students catching TB led to the passage of a 1901 territorial law banning lungers from teaching school in New Mexico. Despite this law, some lungers convinced doctors to conceal their illness. By 1937, a survey of 3,352 students showed a high percentage of pupils with TB. The death rate from TB was considerably higher among Hispanics than among Anglos. (Courtesy of the University of New Mexico Archives.)

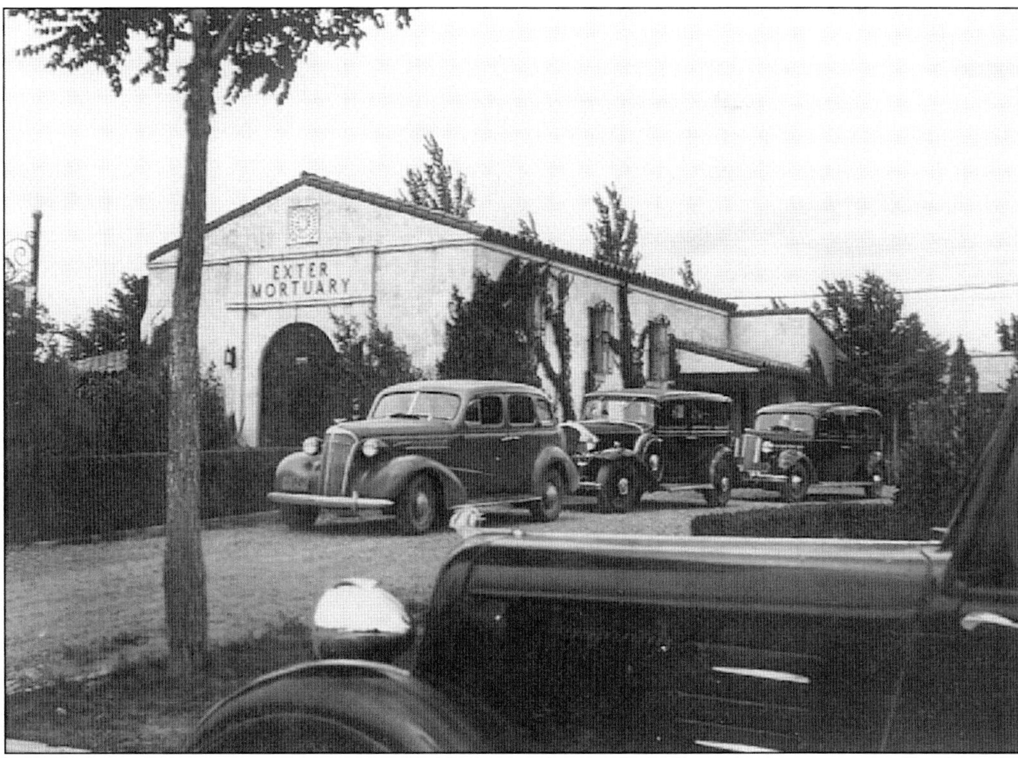

Funeral homes befriended lungers in various ways. Much of what they did was out of kindness, although their more mercenary purpose was to ensure future business. Patients often indicated which funeral director they preferred if they succumbed to TB. Referring to O.W. Strong's funeral home in Albuquerque, Anne Ellis quoted a fellow lunger as saying, "Well, Ellis, if we don't get well, we'll sure get Strong." (Courtesy of the Albuquerque Museum, PA2013.003.012.)

Ten

Passing of an Era

The rapid expansion of the TB industry in the 1910s and 1920s was matched by an equally rapid decline in the 1930s and 1940s. The Great Depression eliminated several vulnerable sans that had barely survived the sounder 1920s. Entire sans were listed for sale in Albuquerque's *Health City Sun*. Some small structures were abandoned and demolished. Others were remodeled for new uses, from schools to drug and alcohol rehabilitation centers. Some "cure cottages" are still used as small homes. One former sanatorium is now an apartment complex; another once served as a minimum security prison for women. At least two sans, Fort Bayard and Fort Stanton, are listed in the National Register of Historic Places. Great efforts have been made to honor the forts' past, including with annual events that have drawn thousands of visitors. Only stronger sans survived as medical centers, largely because they had broadened their missions to become general hospitals before, during, or shortly after the Great Depression.

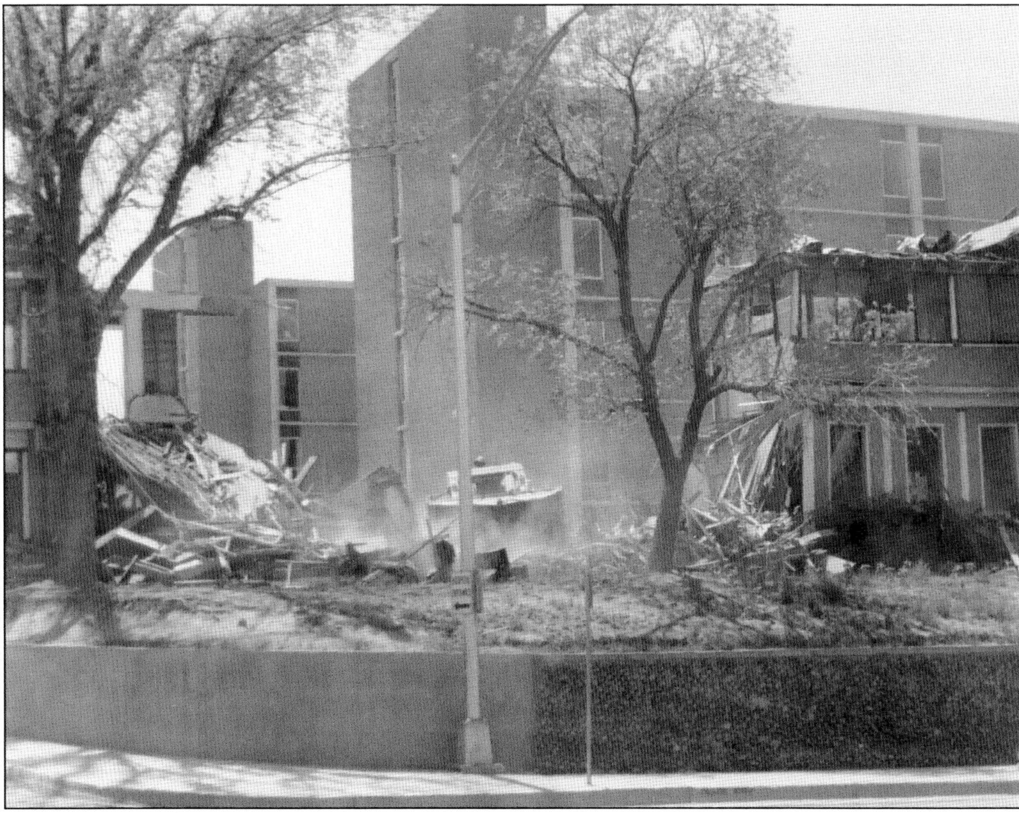

Albuquerque's Presbyterian, St. Joseph (now defunct), and Methodist (now Lovelace); Roswell's St. Mary's; and Santa Fe's Christus St. Vincent's (shown below) are good examples of medical institutions that survived long after their years of service as sanatoriums had passed. Each of these former sans made the transition to a new mission, addressing modern health-care needs. Sans that did not make such a shift usually closed, becoming victims of wrecking balls and urban renewal. The above photograph shows a building in Presbyterian's old san being demolished in 1967, making room for new hospital buildings, some of which are seen in the background. (Above, courtesy of Presbyterian Healthcare Services.)

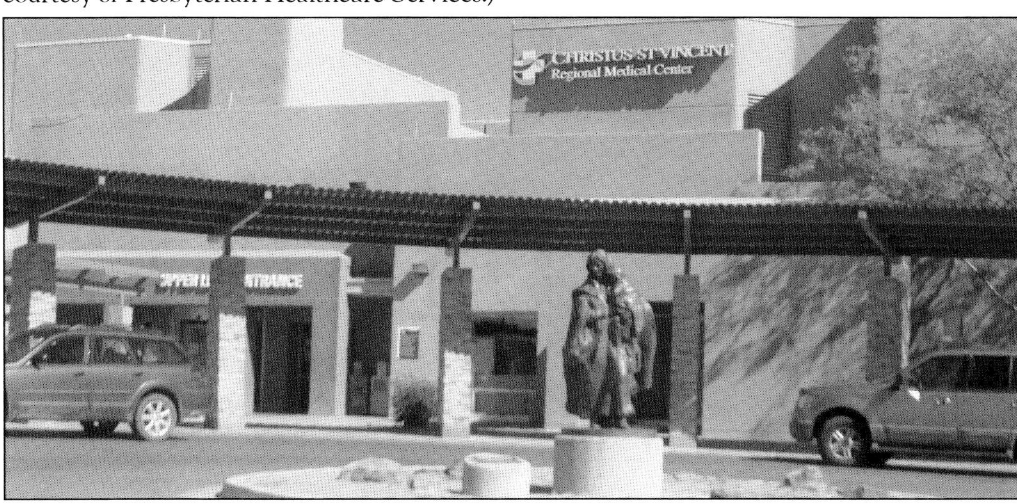

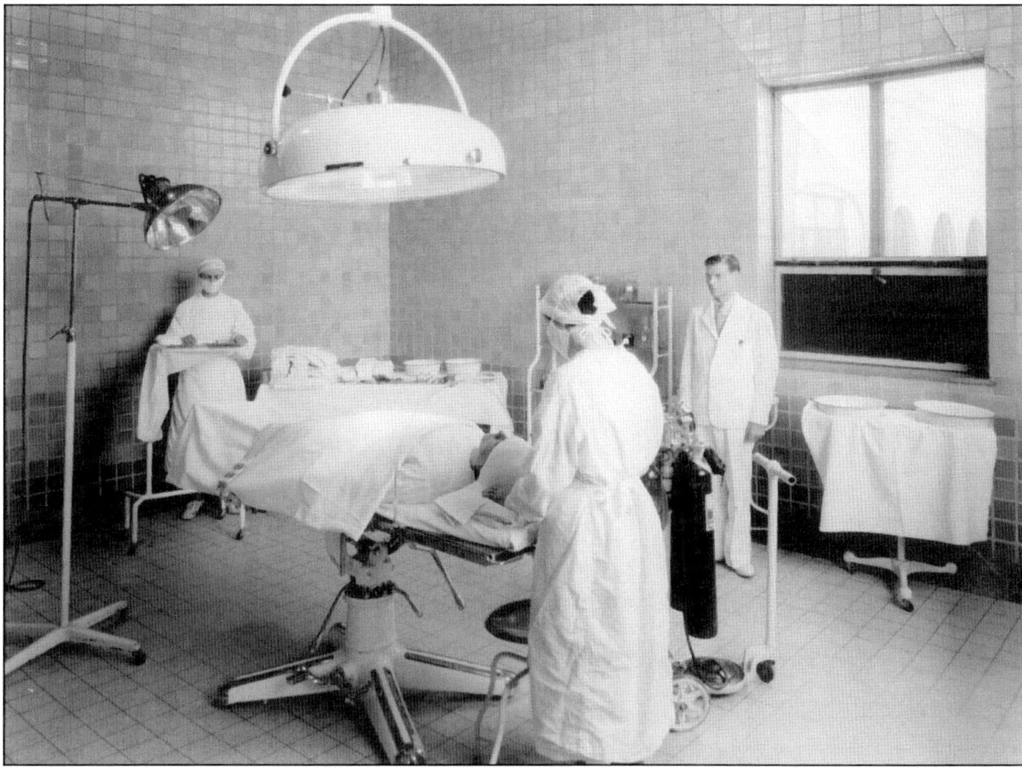

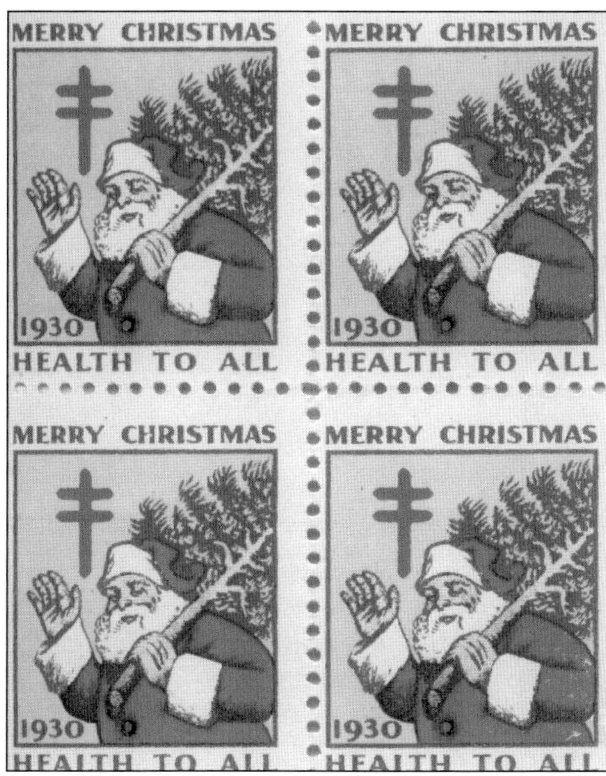

Sanatoriums also closed with the use of surgical procedures and the discovery of effective new drugs. Physicians collapsed or artificially inflated patients' lungs, giving diseased lungs periods of prolonged rest and, hopefully, healing. Both procedures required rest, but rest that could be taken in almost any place, in almost any climate. Years of medical research, funded largely by the sale of Christmas Seals, finally produced promising results. The discovery of streptomycin in 1944 and other new drugs in the early 1950s all but eliminated TB and the need for the unique institutions that had specialized in its treatment for so long in American—and New Mexico—history. (Above, courtesy of Presbyterian Healthcare Services.)